Critical Care Nursing
REVIEW

Second Edition

William G. Gossman
Scott H. Plantz
Sheryl L. Gossman
Roger Skebelsky
Brent Grady
Nicholas Lorenzo

McGraw-Hill
Medical Publishing Division

New York Chicago San Francisco Lisbon London
Madrid Mexico City Milan New Delhi
San Juan Seoul Singapore
Sydney Toronto

The McGraw·Hill Companies

Critical Care Nursing Review, Second Edition

4 5 6 7 8 9 0   CUS/CUS   0 9 8

ISBN 0-07-146423-9

Notice

Medicine is an ever-changing science. As new research and clinical experience broaden our knowledge, changes in treatment and drug therapy are required. The authors and the publisher of this work have checked with sources believed to be reliable in their efforts to provide information that is complete and generally in accord with the standards accepted at the time of publication. However, in view of the possibility of human error or changes in medical sciences, neither the authors nor the publisher nor any other party who has been involved in the preparation or publication of this work warrants that the information contained herein is in every respect accurate or complete, and they disclaim all responsibility for any errors or omissions or for the results obtained from use of the information contained in this work. Readers are encouraged to confirm the information contained herein with other sources. For example and in particular, readers are advised to check the product information sheet included in the package of each drug they plan to administer to be certain that the information contained in this work is accurate and that changes have not been made in the recommended dose or in the contraindications for administration. This recommendation is of particular importance in connection with new or infrequently used drugs.

The editors were Catherine A. Johnson and Marsha Loeb.
The production supervisor was Phil Galea.
The cover designer was Handel Low.
Von Hoffmann Graphics was printer and binder.

This book is printed on acid-free paper.

Cataloging-in-Publication data for this title is on file at the Library of Congress.

DEDICATION

To our little ladies Casey and Taylor.

Bill & Sherry

To my wife Cynna for giving meaning to my life.

Scott

To my family

Roger

To my daughter Chelsey

Brent

To my wife Anne, my son Adam, and to my wonderful parents.

Nick

EDITORS

William G. Gossman, M.D.
Assistant Professor
Finch University/Chicago Medical School
Project Medical Director
Mount Sinai Hospital
Chicago, IL

Scott H. Plantz, M.D.
Associate Professor
Chicago Medical School
Mt. Sinai Medical Center
Chicago, IL

FIRST EDITION CONTRIBUTORS

Sheryl L. Gossman, RN, BSN
Naperville, IL

Roger Skebelsky, PA-C, BSN, RN
Department of Emergency Medicine
Mount Sinai Hospital
Chicago, IL

Brent Grady, RN, CCRN, CEN
Flight Nurse
Loyola Hospital
Maywood, IL

Nicholas Lorenzo, M.D.
Neurology Consultants
Papillion, NE
Bayway Medical Services
St. Petersburg, FL

Kwesi Hankins, RN
Department of Emergency Medicine
Methodist Hospital
Peoria, IL

Brian Murphy, RN
Critical Care Department
Little Company of Mary Hospital
Evergreen Park, IL

Kristine Wengel, RN, BSN, CCRN
Surgical Critical Care Unit
Rush-Presbyterian-St. Luke's Medical Center
Chicago, IL

Marilyn L. Yucaitis, RNBA, CEN, TNCCP, ENPC
Department of Emergency Medicine
Mount Sinai Hospital
Chicago, IL

Bobby Abrams, M.D., FAAEM
Attending Physician
Macomb Hospital
Macomb, MI

Jonathan Adler, M.D., FAAEM
Assistant in Emergency Medicine,
Massachusetts General Hospital
Instructor in Medicine,
Harvard Medical School
Boston, MA

James W. Albers, M.D., Ph.D.
Department of Neurology
University of Michigan
Ann Arbor, MI

Linda Anderson, M.D.
Department of Internal Medicine
Pulmonary and Critical Care Medicine Section
University of Nebraska Medical Center
Omaha, NE

Michael L. Ault, M.D.
Section of Critical Care Medicine
Department of Anesthesiology
Northwestern University Medical School
Chicago, IL

Brian Bonanni, M.D.
Duke University Medical Center
Durham, NC

Jon M. Braverman, M.D.
Denver Health Medical Center
University of Colorado School of Medicine
Denver, CO

David F. M. Brown, M.D.
Instructor in Medicine
Harvard Medical School
Massachusetts General Hospital
Boston, MA

Edward Buckley, M.D.
Department of Neurology
Duke University Medical Center
Durham, NC

Eduardo Castro, M.D.
Instructor in Medicine
Harvard Medical School
Massachusetts General Hospital
Boston, MA

Seemant Chatruvedi, M.D.
Assistant Professor of Neurology
Wayne State University School of medicine
Detroit, MI

Ronald D. Chervin, M.D., MS
Department of Neurology
University of Michigan Health System
Ann Arbor, MI

David Chiu, M.D.
Assistant Professor of Neurology
Baylor College of Medicine
The Methodist Hospital
Houston, TX

Charles H. Cook, M.D.
Assistant Professor of Surgery and Critical Care
The Ohio State University Hospitals
Columbus, OH

Joseph T. Cooke, M.D., FACCP
Associate Professor of Clinical Medicine
Associate Director, Medical Critical Care
The New York Hospital-Cornell Medical Center
New York, NY

C. James Corrall, M.D., MPH
Clinical Associate Professor of Pediatrics
Clinical Associate Professor of EM
Indiana University School of Medicine
Indianapolis, IN

G. Paul Dabrowski, M.D.
Assistant Professor of Surgery
University of Pennsylvania
Philadelphia, PA

Brian J. Daley, M.D.
Assistant Professor
Division of Trauma and Critical Care
The University of Tennessee Medical Center
Knoxville, TN

Joshua De Leon, M.D.
Assistant Professor of Medicine
Mount Sinai School of Medicine
New York, NY

Peter Emblad, M.D.
Boston City Hospital
Boston, MA

Phillip Fairweather, M.D.
Clinical Assistant Professor
Mount Sinai School of Medicine
New York, NY
Department of Emergency Medicine
Elmhurst Hospital Center
Elmhurst, NY

Craig Feied, M.D.
Clinical Associate Professor
George Washington University
Washington Hospital Center
Washington, D.C.

Eva L. Feldman, M.D., Ph.D.
Department of Neurology
University of Michigan
Ann Arbor, MI

Louis Flancbaum, M.D., FACS, FCCM, FCCP
Associate Professor of Surgery, Anesthesiology,
and Human Nutrition
The Ohio State University Hospitals
Columbus, OH

Mark Franklin, M.D.
Department of Anesthesiology
Northwestern University Medical School
Chicago, IL

Rajesh R. Gandhi, M.D.
Critical Care/Trauma Fellow
University of Pennsylvania
Philadelphia, PA

Vicente H. Gracias, M.D.
Instructor of Surgery and Trauma
Surgical Critical Care Fellow
University of Pennsylvania
Philadelphia, PA

L. John Greenfield, Jr., M.D., Ph.D.
Assistant Professor
Department of Neurology
University of Michigan
Ann Arbor, MI

Susan M. Harding, M.D.
Assistant Professor of Medicine
Pulmonary and Critical Care Medicine
University of Alabama
Birmingham, AL

James F. Holmes, M.D.
University of California, Davis
School of Medicine
Sacramento, CA

Eddie Hooker, M.D.
Assistant Professor
University of Louisville
Louisville, KY

Cameron Javid, M.D.
Department of Ophthalmology
Tulane University
New Orleans, LA

Mishith Joshi, M.D.
Department of Neurology
Wayne State University
Detroit, MI

Marc J. Kahn, M.D.
Assistant Professor of Medicine
Tulane University School of Medicine
New Orleans, LA

Henry J. Kaminski, M.D.
Case Western Reserve University School of
Medicine
Department of Veterans Affairs Medical Center
University Hospitals of Cleveland
Cleveland, OH

Stuart Kessler, M.D.
Vice Chairman, Department of Emergency
Medicine
Mount Sinai School of Medicine
New York, NY
Director, Department of Emergency Medicine
Elmhurst Hospital Center
Elmhurst, NY

Lance W. Kreplick, M.D.
Assistant Professor
University of Illinois
EHS Christ Hospital
Oak Lawn, IL

Andrew Lee, M.D.
Department of Ophthalmology
Baylor College of Medicine
Houston, TX

Richard Lenhardt, M.D.
Harvard Medical School
Boston, MA

Joseph Lieber, M.D.
Associate Attending in Medicine
Elmhurst Hospital Center
Clinical Associate Professor of Medicine
Mount Sinai School of Medicine
New York, NY

Bernard Lopez, M.D.
Assistant Professor
Thomas Jefferson Medical College
Thomas Jefferson University Hospital
Philadelphia, PA

Kenneth Maiese, M.D.
Associate Professor
Departments of Neurology and Anatomy & Cell
Biology
Wayne State University School of Medicine
Detroit, MI

John T. Malcynski, M.D.
Instructor of Surgery and Trauma
Surgical Critical Care Fellow
University of Pennsylvania
Philadelphia, PA

Mary Nan S. Mallory, M.D.
University of Louisville
Louisville, KY

Gregory P. Marelich, M.D., FACP, FCCP
Assistant Professor of Clinical Internal Medicine
Division of Pulmonary and Critical Care
Medicine
University of California Davis Medical Center
Sacramento, CA

Terence McGarry, M.D.
Pulmonary and Critical Care Medicine
Elmhurst Hospital Center
Elmhurst, NY
Assistant Professor of Medicine
Mount Sinai School of Medicine
New York, NY

David Morgan, M.D.
University of Texas
Southwestern Medical Center
Parkland Memorial Hospital
Dallas, TX

Gholam K. Motamedi, M.D.
Department of Neurology
Baylor College of Medicine
Houston, TX

Anthony M. Murro, M.D.
Associate Professor of Neurology
Medical College of Georgia
Augusta, GA

Debra Myers, M.D.
Assistant Professor
Department of Internal medicine
Wayne State University School of Medicine
Detroit, MI

Sarah T. Nath, M.D.
Sleep Disorders Center
Department of Neurology
University of Michigan Health System
Ann Arbor, MI

Lavi Oud, M.D.
Department of Critical Care Medicine
Wayne State University School of Medicine
Detroit, MI

Deric M. Park, M.D.
Department of Neurology
The University of Chicago
Chicago, IL

Scott H. Plantz, M.D., FAAEM
Assistant Professor
Chicago Medical School
Sinai Medical Center
Chicago, IL

Anthony T. Reder, M.D.
Associate Professor of Neurology
Department of Neurology
The University of Chicago
Chicago, IL

Juan Carlos Restrepo, M.D.
Diplomat of the American Board of
Anesthesiology
Board Certified in Critical Care Medicine
VA Medical Center – Jackson Memorial
Hospital
University of Miami
Miami, FL

Lisa Rogers, D.O.
Associate Professor of Neurology
Wayne State University School of Medicine
Detroit, MI

Carlo Rosen, M.D.
Instructor in Medicine
Harvard Medical School
Massachusetts General Hospital
Boston, MA

James A. Rowley, M.D.
Assistant Professor of Medicine
Division of Pulmonary/Critical Care Medicine
Wayne State University School of Medicine
Detroit, MI

Bruce K. Rubin, M.D.
Professor of Pediatrics, Physiology and
Pharmacology
Brenner Children's Hospital
Winston-Salem, NC

David Rubenstein, M.D.
Division of Cardiology
Elmhurst Hospital Center
Elmhurst, NY

Robert L. Ruff, M.D., Ph.D.
Departments of Neurology and Neurosciences
Case Western Reserve University School of
Medicine
Department of Veterans Affairs Medical Center
University Hospitals of Cleveland
Cleveland, OH

Nelson R. Sabates, M.D.
Eye Foundation of Kansas City
University of Missouri, Kansas City School of
Medicine
Kansas City, MO

Harvey M. Shanies, Ph.D., M.D.
Clinical Associate Professor of Medicine
Mount Sinai School of Medicine
New York, NY
Associate Director of Critical Care Medicine
Elmhurst Hospital Center
Elmhurst, NY

Arunabh Sharma, M.D.
Fellow in Pulmonary and Critical Care Medicine
Brigham and Women's Hospital
Havard Medical School
Boston, MA

Anders A.F. Sima, M.D., Ph.D.
Professor of Pathology and Neurology
Wayne State University School of Medicine
Detroit, MI

Giles Simpson, M.D.
Assistant Professor of Emergency Medicine
Mount Sinai Hospital
Chicago, IL

Sabine Sobek, M.D.
Department of Critical Care Medicine
Wayne State University School of Medicine
Detroit, MI

Dana Stearns, M.D.
Instructor in Medicine
Harvard Medical School
Massachusetts General Hospital
Boston, MA

Jack Stump, M.D.
Attending Physician
Rogue Valley Medical Center
Medford, OR

Joan Surdukowski, M.D.
Assistant Professor
Chicago Medical School
Mt. Sinai Hospital
Chicago, IL

Menno Terriet, M.D.
Department of Anesthesia
Veterans Affairs Medical Center
Miami, FL

Carlo Tornatore, M.D.
Assistant Professor of Neurology
Georgetown University Medical Center
Washington, DC

Mythili Venkataraman, M.D.
Attending, Pulmonary Medicine
Assistant Professor of Medicine
Mount Sinai School of Medicine
New York, NY

Mladen Vidovich, M.D.
Department of Anesthesiology
Northwestern University Medical School
Chicago, IL

Martin Warshawsky, M.D., FACP, FCCP
Director, Respiratory Intensive Care Unit
Assistant Professor of Medicine
Mount Sinai School of Medicine
New York, NY

Mike Zevitz, M.D.
Assistant Professor
Chicago Medical School
Chicago, IL

INTRODUCTION

Congratulations! *Critical Care Nursing Review: Pearls of Wisdom* will help you learn about critical care medicine as well as prepare for the critical care board examination. This book is structured in a question and answer format. It is useful as a self-assessment while studying for the critical care exam. This permits the reader to concentrate on areas of interest or weakness. Some readers will find answering questions the preferred way to study for a board exam. After completing a chapter, readers are encouraged to examine the corresponding textbook chapter entirely, for comprehensiveness.

Most readers will probably use this book in a post-textbook review mode. One such method involves reading a chapter in a textbook then proceeding to answer the questions posed in this book. Other readers will prefer to comprehensively study the contents of critical care medicine entirely and use this book afterwards. The purpose of the last two methods is to permit the reader to uncover areas of weakness and to become familiarized with the process of answering questions. Answering questions during a board exam is a cognitive task that is optimized by preparing a specific set of cognitive skills.

It must be emphasized that a question and answer book is most useful as a learning tool when used in conjunction with a textbook of critical care medicine. This is because the question/answer format is an active learning process that is at its best when the questioning process continues farther along than ending with answering the *Critical Care Nursing Review* question. The more active the learning process, the better the understanding. When the reader approaches a question that he/she cannot recall the answer to or uncovers a topic of interest, he/she is encouraged to read in the textbook at hand.

Most of the questions are short with short answers. This facilitates moving through a large body of knowledge. Some of the questions have longer answers. In these situations, the questions were not altered because of the clinically interesting question posed.

The chapters are organized to include all aspects of critical care medicine. The questions within each chapter are randomly presented, to simulate board exams and the way questions arise in real life. Certain topics have been repeated in a single chapter and across chapters. This was intentional because some topics are so important that redundancy is used to help you master that topic. Each question is preceded by a hollow bullet, to permit the reader to check off areas of interest or weakness, or simply noting that it had been read. This allows for re-reading without having uncertainty of what was reviewed earlier.

Great effort has been made to verify that the questions and answers are accurate. Some answers may not be the answer you would prefer. Most often this is attributable to variance between original sources. Please make us aware of any errors you find. We hope to make continuous improvements and would greatly appreciate any input with regard to format, organization, content, presentation or about specific questions. We also are interested in recruiting new contributing authors and publishing new textbooks. We look forward to hearing form you!

Study hard and good luck!

W.G.G., S.H.P., S.L.G., R.S., B.G., N.L.

TABLE OF CONTENTS

AIRWAY, RESUSCITATION AND VENTILATOR PEARLS

O   **What is the benefit to rapid sequence induction in the emergency setting?**

The use of a paralytic agent, as succinylcholine, enhances the ease of intubation and prevents aspiration by paralyzing the muscles. Paralytic agents should not be used without agents that induce unconsciousness.

O   **In a trauma patient with multiple fractures, internal injuries and an unstable airway, emergent endotracheal intubation in the emergency department is considered prior to definitive surgical therapy.   What are the most likely hemodynamic consequences of intubation and initiation of mechanical ventilation in this subject?**

Hypotension may occur during or following endotracheal intubation and the institution of positive pressure ventilation. This cardiovascular decompensation is due to a decrease in venous return associated with both the use of sympatholytic agents for induction and the positive pressure induced increase in intrathoracic pressure.

O   **What is the average distance from the external nares to the carina in males and females?**

32 cm and 27 cm, respectively.

O   **How long should a patient be preoxygenated to achieve a denitrogenation level such that apnea for 3 to 5 minutes maintains the oxygen saturation above 90%?**

5 minutes in the normal individual.

O   **What is the mean average rise of carbon dioxide in apneic oxygenation?**

3 mmHg/min.

O   **T/F: Too much lidocaine may cause seizures.**

True.

O   **What is the safest technique to intubate a child with epiglottitis?**

Intubation in the operating room after induction of anesthesia with an inhaled anesthetic (halothane or sevoflurane) in the semi-sitting position.

O   **What is the incidence of impossible mask ventilation?**

1 in 5000 anesthetics.

O   **At what peak inspiratory pressure should an air leak be detected in pediatric patients intubated with an appropriate sized endotracheal tube?**

25 to 30 cm H_2O.

O   **What is the most common cause of upper airway obstruction?**

The tongue occluding the posterior oropharynx.

O   **Name some important adjuncts often needed to help establish basic airway control.**

Suction equipment to remove secretions from mouth and throat, chin lift-jaw thrust maneuver, oral/nasal airway and bag-valve-mask device.

O   **What are some advanced techniques for airway management?**

Orotracheal intubation, nasotracheal intubation, esophageal obturator airway (EOA), esophageal gastric tube airway (EGTA), pharyngotracheal airway, combination esophageal-tracheal tube, cricothyroidotomy and tracheostomy.

O   **What are some indications for intubation?**

Apnea, burns, acute airway obstruction, expanding neck hematomas, hemodynamic instability, severe head injuries, poor oxygenation, poor ventilation, prevention of aspiration, inability to maintain a patent airway and impending or potential compromise of the airway.

O   **What must be kept in mind when performing endotracheal intubation in a trauma patient?**

The potential for cervical spine injury.

O   **What is a potential problem with bag-valve-mask ventilation?**

Air can enter the stomach via the esophagus causing gastric distention and aspiration.

O   **How many people does it take to effectively ventilate a patient via the bag-valve-mask technique?**

Two. One to hold the mask securely to the face and a second to squeeze the bag with two hands.

O   **Does tracheal intubation prevent aspiration?**

No. Microaspiration can still occur.

O   **What characteristic of gastric contents causes the greatest harm following aspiration?**

Although particulate matter can clog the airways leading to atelectasis, it is the acidity of the gastric contents that leads to the greatest injury.

O   **Name some factors that place a patient at risk for aspiration.**

Full stomach, trauma, intra-abdominal pathology (obstruction, inflammation, gastric paresis), esophageal disease (symptomatic reflux, motility disorders), pregnancy and obesity.

O   **What properties of succinylcholine make it particularly useful as an aid for intubation?**

Succinylcholine, a depolarizing paralytic agent, has a brief duration of action (3 to 5 minutes) and a rapid onset of action (within 60 seconds).

❍ **What are the possible deleterious effects of succinylcholine?**

Increased intragastric, intraocular and intracranial pressure.
Hyperkalemia, particularly in neurologic and burn injuries.
Increased duration of action in the rare patient with pseudocholinesterase deficiency.

❍ **What equipment is needed to assist with endotracheal intubation?**

Suction for the mouth and pharynx, bag-valve-mask system for oxygenation, functioning laryngoscope, stylet and endotracheal tubes.

❍ **In the typical male patient, what length of ET tube should lay distal to the lips?**

23 cm.

❍ **In the typical female patient, what length of ET tube should lay distal to the lips?**

21 cm.

❍ **What is the consequence of an ET tube placed too far distally?**

Respiratory insufficiency secondary to right mainstem bronchus intubation.

❍ **How is right mainstem intubation diagnosed?**

Decreased breath sounds on the left that corrects with repositioning of the ET tube.

❍ **What type of endotracheal tube cuff is presently used?**

High-volume, low pressure cuffs. (Pressure = 20 to 25 mmHg.)

❍ **When does tracheal ischemia occur?**

When the pressure in the endotracheal tube cuff exceeds capillary perfusion pressure (typically 25 to 35 mmHg).

❍ **Immediately after inserting an ET tube, what is the next most appropriate step?**

Confirm tube placement.

❍ **How is proper endotracheal tube placement confirmed?**

Symmetric chest expansion, breath sounds in axillae but not over the epigastrium, tube fogs with respirations, end-tidal CO_2, monitoring of oxygen saturation and visualizing the tube passing through the vocal cords.

❍ **Does a chest x-ray guarantee correct endotracheal tube placement?**

No. Clinical signs (see last question) are needed for confirmation of endotracheal tube placement.

❍ **What is the correct position of the tip of the endotracheal tube?**

Approximately 4 cm above the carina.

○   **What is the most common complication of nasotracheal intubation?**

Epistaxis.

○   **What are the signs of tension pneumothorax on physical exam?**

Tachypnea, unilateral absent breath sounds, tachycardia, pallor, diaphoresis, cyanosis, tracheal deviation, hypotension and neck vein distention.

○   **What determines the relationship between changes in airway pressure and lung volume during positive pressure ventilation?**

Lung and chest wall compliance combine to define the relation between airway pressure and lung volume. Increased stiffness of the lungs (pulmonary fibrosis or overdistention) or the chest wall (obesity) will decrease the amount to which lung volume will increase for a given increase in airway pressure.

○   **A young male patient awaiting general anesthesia is found to have a heart rate of 60 beats per minute which increases up to about 80 beats per minute with each spontaneous inspiration. What is this patient's condition?**

He is normal. Healthy young adults normally have a relative bradycardia and normal inspiration induces an in-phase vagal withdrawal that causes heart rate to increase during inspiration and decrease during expiration. This phenomenon is referred to as respiratory sinus arrhythmia.

○   **In a diabetic patient breathing spontaneously prior to induction of general anesthesia, the physician noted that the baseline heart rate was 88 beats per minute but that there was no discernible heart rate variability on the cardiac monitor, suggesting the absence of respiratory sinus arrhythmia. Is this a problem?**

Potentially yes. Absence of normal respiratory sinus arrhythmia infers dysautonomia. The patient is at increased risk of systemic hypotension following induction of general anesthesia because the normal adaptive autonomic responses may also be absent.

○   **Acute elevations in pulmonary arterial pressure do what to left ventricular diastolic compliance?**

It is decreased because of interventricular dependence of the left and right ventricles.

○   **How does spontaneous ventilation, by inducing negative swings in intrathoracic pressure, affect myocardial oxygen demand?**

It is increased becaues of increased left ventricular afterload.

○   **Under normal conditions at rest, what percentage of the cardiac output goes to the respiratory muscles?**

Less than 3%.

○   **In patients with COPD, what percentage of the total cardiac output may be directed to the muscles of respiration?**

25 to 30%.

O   **Positive end-expiratory pressure (PEEP) primarily impairs cardiac output by what mechanism?**

Decrease in LV preload.

O   **To the extent that LV preload is maintained, positive pressure ventilation has what effect on cardiac output in patients with normal cardiovascular function?**

No measurable effect as compared to spontaneous ventilation.

O   **When two different modes of ventilation, such as pressure support and inverse ratio ventilation, have similar changes in intrathoracic pressure and ventilatory effort, how do their hemodynamic effects compare?**

Similar.

O   **Can the hemodynamic effects of mechanical ventilation be seen in non-intubated patients during non-invasive ventilatory support?**

Yes. Identical effects should be seen for the same changes in lung volume and intrathoracic pressure.

O   **Is there any hemodynamic difference between increasing airway pressure to generate a breath and decreasing extrathoracic pressure (iron lung negative pressure ventilation) to generate a similar tidal volume?**

None, if the iron lung encompasses the entire body. However, if it surrounds only the chest and abdomen, it may have less detrimental effects due to the sparing of venous return.

O   **Weaning from mechanical ventilation is associated with what effect on myocardial oxygen demand?**

Increased MVO_2. Consider weaning to be a cardiac stress test.

O   **In patients with congestive heart failure, cardiovascular insufficiency and respiratory distress, the initiation of positive pressure ventilation is often associated with what hemodynamic response?**

Improvement in overall cardiovascular status due to the combined effects of the associated reduced work of breathing and reduced LV afterload.

O   **In patients with unilateral lung injury, is the effect of positive end-expiratory pressure applied at the trachea the same as in patients with bilateral lung injury?**

No. PEEP may overdistend the healthy lung in subjects with unilateral lung injury causing an increase in the amount of intrapulmonary shunt and pulmonary vascular resistance.

O   **An intubated patient with ischemic heart disease develops mild inspiratory stridor upon extubation associated with severe chest pain and marked ST segment elevations across the precordium. The immediate treatment of this condition should include what ventilatory therapy?**

Eliminate the markedly negative swings in intrathoracic pressure by re-intubation.

O   **In a patient with acute lung injury breathing spontaneously, intubation and the application of both an enriched FIO$_2$ and PEEP sufficient to recruit collapsed alveolar units should do what to pulmonary vascular resistance?**

Decrease it by reversing hypoxic pulmonary vasoconstriction.

O   **A mechanically ventilated patient with chronic obstructive lung disease is breathing spontaneously on assist-control mode with a measured intrinsic PEEP of 12 cm H$_2$O. What will the application of 8 cm H$_2$O extrinsic PEEP (from the ventilatory circuit) do to the patient's work of breathing?**

In general it will decrease the work of breathing by reducing the amount of airway pressure drop needed to trigger the positive pressure breath. Some patients with intrinsic PEEP may have deleterious effect when adding PEEP to the ventilator circuit. Careful monitoring of the patient is mandatory. The level of added PEEP should be less than the amount of intrinsic PEEP.

O   **What is peripheral cyanosis?**

Peripheral cyanosis is due to shunting or increased O$_2$ extraction.

O   **Name the two primary causes (groups) of peripheral cyanosis.**

Cyanosis with a normal SaO$_2$ can be due to:
     Decreased cardiac output.
     Redistribution - may be 2° to shock, DIC, hypothermia, vascular obstruction.

O   **What is heliox and when is it used?**

Helium has less density than oxygen and is thought to decrease the turbulence of flow past sites of obstruction. Heliox is a combination of helium and oxygen that is used when patients have an upper airway obstruction to decrease stridor, increase tidal volume and improve ventilation.

O   **What disorders are associated with auto-PEEP?**

Asthma, COPD and ARDS.

O   **What are the pulmonary criteria for extubation?**

Tidal volume of at least 5 ml/kg, vital capacity of 15 ml/kg, negative inspiratory force less than -25 cm H$_2$O, respiratory rate greater than 10 and less than 30, adequate oxygenation on an inspired oxygen concentration of 40% or less, ratio of spontaneous breathing frequency to tidal volume (in liters) less than 100, ability to protect the airway, and no excessive secretions.

O   **Which patients are at risk for developing aspiration pneumonia?**

Patients undergoing emergency surgery, pregnant patients, obese patients, those with gastrointestinal obstruction, depressed level of consciousness and laryngeal incompetence.

O   **What is the appropriate treatment following aspiration?**

Secure the airway, administer oxygen, suction any aspirate, consider bronchoscopy if large particulates are present, ventilatory support and bronchodilators as needed for bronchospasm.

O   A patient is admitted to the SICU after surgical debridement for necrotizing pancreatitis. Over the next several hours, the patient's oxygenation deteriorates, with oxygen saturation of 90% on 75% inspired oxygen and 10 of PEEP. What is the most likely diagnosis?

ARDS.

O   T/F: Acute lung injury of the entire lung causes lung compliance to decrease similarly in each region of the lung.

False. Marked regional differences in the degree of lung consolidation and compliance characterize all forms of acute lung injury.

O   How does positive pressure ventilation increase the cardiac output in patients with a low left ventricular ejection fraction?

Decreased afterload.

O   What are the determinants of $PaCO_2$?

Carbon dioxide production and alveolar ventilation.

O   What are the components of tidal volume?

Alveolar volume and dead space volume.

O   What is the maximum acceptable endotracheal tube cuff pressure?

Approximately 25 cm H_2O at the end of expiration.

O   What is the potential harm of excess endotracheal tube cuff pressure?

It can induce ischemia and necrosis of the underlying tissue.

O   Adequacy of alveolar ventilation is reflected by which component of arterial blood gas analysis?

$PaCO_2$.

O $PaCO_2$ is mathematically related to alveolar ventilation in what manner?

Inverse proportion.

O   What factors interfere with the bellows function of the chest?

Abdominal binding, massive obesity, trauma with flail chest, massive effusion and ascites, pneumothorax, thoracic burn with eschar, neuromuscular blockade and strapping of ribs.

O   How does malnutrition contribute to respiratory failure?

Respiratory muscle weakness.

O   Respiratory failure is worsened in spinal injuries at or above which nerve root?

C2.

○ **What infectious syndromes can lead to ventilatory insufficiency?**

Botulism, tetanus, campylobacter, polio, diphtheria and Guillain-Barre Syndrome.

○ **T/F: Pulmonary capillary wedge pressure (PCWP) is a reflection of left atrial pressure.**

True.

○ **What processes cause the work of breathing to increase markedly in patients with COPD?**

Increased dead space ventilation, decreased respiratory muscle efficiency and increased airway resistance.

○ **What are the most common causes of increased dead space in critically ill patients?**

Decreased cardiac output, pulmonary embolism, pulmonary hypertension, ARDS and excessive PEEP.

○ **The total work of breathing is divided into what two parts?**

Overcoming lung and chest wall compliance and overcoming airway resistance.

○ **Blood drawn from the tip of a pulmonary artery catheter wedged in zone III will reflect PO_2 from what source?**

Pulmonary capillary.

○ **Which mitral valve abnormalities can lead to large v waves on the pulmonary artery wedge tracing?**

Both mitral stenosis and mitral regurgitation because of overfilling of the left atrium.

○ **What is the hemodynamic response to an acute complete spinal cord injury at the C7 level?**

Initially there is hypertension and tachycardia secondary to increased circulating catecholamines at the time of the injury followed shortly by hypotension due to vasodilatation and bradycardia secondary to loss of cardiac accelerator input.

○ **During the first minute of apnea, how much would you expect the $PaCO_2$ to rise?**

During apnea, the $PaCO_2$ will increase approximately 6 mmHg during the first minute and then 3 to 4 mmHg each minute thereafter.

○ **What is the most important factor in control of ventilation under normal conditions?**

Arterial $PaCO_2$.

○ **What is functional residual capacity (FRC)?**

The volume of gas in the lung after a normal expiration is the FRC and is comprised of residual volume and expiratory reserve volume.

❍ **What are the major causes of arterial hypoxemia?**

Hypoventilation, ventilation/perfusion inequality, shunt, low FIO_2 and diffusion impairment.

❍ **How does one assess oxygenation?**

Skin color, pulse oximetry and blood gas analysis.

❍ **How does one assess ventilation?**

End tidal CO_2 monitoring and blood gas analysis.

❍ **What is a tension pneumothorax?**

An injury to the lung allowing intrapleural air to collect without escaping via the chest wall or trachea. This accumulation of air compresses the lung and shifts the mediastinum, leading to impaired venous return and hypotension.

❍ **What are the physical findings in tension pneumothorax?**

Distended neck veins, hypotension, tracheal deviation and a hyperresonant hemithorax.

❍ **What is the treatment for tension pneumothorax?**

Immediate needle decompression of the hyperresonant hemithorax, based on clinical suspicion. Radiography should not be used to confirm tension pneumothorax.

❍ **What is adequate urinary output to gauge resuscitation in adults?**

0.5 cc/kg or about 50 cc/hr.

❍ **What effect does intrinsic PEEP have on the work of breathing in patients receiving mechanical ventilation?**

Increased elastic work and increased work to trigger assisted breaths.

❍ **How can the work of breathing with mechanical ventilation associated with intrinsic PEEP be reduced?**

Add a small amount of PEEP, reduce tidal volume, reduce inspiratory time and increase expiratory time.

❍ **What complications are associated with mask ventilation?**

Skin breakdown, aspiration pneumonia, aerophagia, pneumothorax and barotrauma (volutrauma).

❍ **Through what mechanism does PEEP decrease cardiac output?**

Reduced preload.

❍ **What evidence of barotrauma can be observed on chest x-ray?**

Pneumomediastinum, pneumothorax, pneumopericardium, subcutaneous emphysema and pulmonary interstitial emphysema.

○   **What are the primary determinants of the work of breathing?**

Minute ventilation, lung/chest wall compliance, airway resistance and presence of intrinsic PEEP.

○   **What are some conditions under which CO_2 production is increased?**

Lipogenesis, fever and hyperthyroidism.

○   **What is the preferred FIO_2 for patients with ARDS?**

The lowest that will maintain a hemoglobin oxygen saturation of about 90%.

○   **What is the primary determinant of the oxygen content of arterial blood?**

The product of hemoglobin concentration and the percent hemoglobin oxygen saturation of arterial blood. The amount of oxygen dissolved in the plasma (a function of the PaO_2) is negligible at one atmosphere of pressure.

○   **How can adequate tidal volume be delivered to a patient undergoing volume cycled mechanical ventilation whose endotracheal tube cuff is failing to maintain an adequate seal (without changing the tube)?**

Increase the mandatory tidal volume.

○   **What are indications for stress ulcer prophylaxis in critically ill patients?**

Mechanical ventilation and coagulopathy.

○   **What combination of medications, often used in the treatment of status asthmaticus requiring mechanical ventilation, may result in prolonged weakness?**

Steroids and neuromuscular blocking agents.

○   **When may end-tidal carbon dioxide detectors prove inaccurate?**

In patients with very low blood flow to the lungs or in those with a large dead space (e.g., following a pulmonary embolism).

○   **What is the most common complication of endotracheal intubation?**

Intubation of a bronchus. Other complications include esophageal intubation, lacerations of the lip, tongue and pharyngeal or tracheal mucosa, resulting in bleeding, hematoma or abscess. Tracheal rupture, avulsion of an arytenoid cartilage, vocal cord injury, pharyngeal-esophageal perforation, intubation of the pyriform sinus, gastric content aspiration, hypertension, tachycardia and arrhythmias may also occur.

○   **What oxygen flow rate is recommended for facemask ventilation?**

At least 5 L/min. Recommended flow is 8 to 10 L/min., which will produce oxygen concentrations as high as 40% to 60%.

O   **What oxygen concentration can be supplied with a facemask and oxygen reservoir?**

6 L/min. provides approximately 60% oxygen concentration and each liter increases the concentration by 10%. 10 L/min. is almost 100%.

O   **What are the four commonly used modes of ventilation?**

Intermittent mandatory ventilation (IMV), pressure support (PS), assist control (AC) and pressure control (PC).

O   **What is the difference between IMV, SIMV and AC? Can you wean a patient using AC?**

IMV provides a given tidal volume at a set respiratory rate. Any breaths initiated by the patient achieve only the tidal volume the patient is able to generate.

In SIMV (synchronized IMV) the ventilator attempts to synchronize the patient's ventilatory effort with an assisted breath. Breaths in excess of the set respiratory rate do not receive assistance from the ventilator.

In AC all tidal volumes whether initiated by the patient or by the ventilator achieve the set tidal volume. Therefore, you cannot wean a patient in the AC mode.

O   **What is the difference between pressure control ventilation and pressure support ventilation?**

In pressure support ventilation, a breath is spontaneously initiated by the patient. The ventilator delivers a flow of gas to reach a target pressure. This flow is maintained until a flow threshold is reached during the decelerating phase of inspiration. At this time expiration begins.

In pressure control ventilation, a patient receives a mechanical breath at a predetermined rate. Once again the ventilator delivers a flow of gas to reach a certain pressure. Unlike pressure support, the ventilator assists the breath until a predetermined time is reached. This is called time-cycling.

In neither mode is the tidal volume controlled. Instead, the tidal volume is determined by pulmonary compliance, duration of inspiration and synchrony between the ventilator and the patient.

O   **Describe the events associated with auto-PEEP.**

Also known as air trapping and intrinsic PEEP (positive end-expiratory pressure), auto-PEEP occurs mostly in patients with asthma, chronic obstructive pulmonary disease and acute respiratory distress syndrome. Auto-PEEP occurs when a patient with lung disease is unable to completely exhale each tidal volume. The accumulation of pressure results in a persistent difference between alveolar pressure and external airway pressure at end expiration. The persistent pressure difference results in continued airflow at end exhalation.

O   **What are the consequences of auto-PEEP?**

Auto-PEEP results in tidal volumes that occur at the upper limit of total lung capacity where compliance is low. Thus higher pressures are required to achieve a given tidal volume and the patient is at increased risk for barotrauma. In a patient who is initiating breaths on the ventilator (e.g., spontaneously breathing with pressure support), auto-PEEP increases the work of breathing. Like extrinsic PEEP, auto-PEEP can compromise cardiac function by decreasing venous return and cardiac output.

O   **An intubated patient is left on 100% oxygen for 20 hours. Describe changes that can be attributed to oxygen toxicity.**

Tracheobronchial irritation (coughing, substernal discomfort), decreased vital capacity, decreased lung compliance, decreased diffusing capacity, decreased tracheal mucus velocity, increased arteriovenous shunting, absorption atelectasis and increased dead space to tidal volume ratio.

○   **A patient has been ventilator dependent for almost four weeks. She appears to be making slow progress in weaning from the ventilator. What are the advantages and disadvantages of undergoing a tracheotomy?**

A tracheotomy may help by decreasing dead space, improving clearance of secretions and improving patient comfort. It also partially restores glottic function. Assuming the patient progresses well, a tracheotomy also offers the potential to be able to verbally communicate and to tolerate oral feedings.

However, a tracheotomy requires the patient to undergo another surgical procedure. It is also associated with the risks of stoma granulation, tracheal erosion, tracheal stenosis and tracheo-innominate fistula.

○   **What ventilator steps can be taken to optimize an ARDS patient's respiratory function?**

Using pressure control to minimize barotrauma, decreasing tidal volume to minimize volutrauma, using inverse ratio ventilation and permissive hypercapnia to maximize inspiration time. None of these strategies have been proven by clinical trials.

○   **What factors shift the oxygen-hemoglobin dissociation curve to the right?**

Acidemia, increased 2,3 DPG and increased temperature.

○   **Define compliance.**

The change in volume divided by the change in distending pressure. Elastic recoil is usually measured in terms of compliance. Compliance measurements can be obtained for the chest, the lung or both together.

○   **What is the predominant stimulus for activation of hypoxic pulmonary vasoconstriction?**

Decreased alveolar oxygen tension.

○   **What factors can potentially contribute to the difficulty in weaning critically ill patients from mechanical ventilation?**

Lack of central ventilatory drive due to encephalopathy, primary myopathy, muscle fatigue or weakness and neuropathy of critical illness.

○   **What is the mechanism of diaphragm dysfunction following open heart surgery?**

Thermal or mechanical injury to the phrenic nerve.

○   **Which neuromuscular and spinal diseases can lead to ventilatory insufficiency?**

Muscular dystrophy, polymyositis, myotonic dystrophy, polyneuritis, Eaton Lambert syndrome, myasthenia gravis, amyotrophic lateral sclerosis, trauma, Guillain-Barré syndrome, multiple sclerosis, Parkinson's Disease and stroke.

○   **Patients on mechanical ventilation can develop hypoventilation based on what pulmonary factors?**

Increased dead space (including length of ventilator circuit proximal to the "Y" piece separating the inspiratory and expiratory limbs), decreased tidal volume, overdistention of lung, air leaks and massive pulmonary embolism.

❍ **Patients with failure of which organs are at increased risk of developing prolonged paralysis following neuromuscular blocker administration?**

Liver and kidney.

❍ **How is the work of breathing affected by patient triggered positive pressure ventilation?**

It can increase, decrease or remain the same.

❍ **How can the presence of intrinsic PEEP be confirmed in patients undergoing mechanical ventilation?**

Just prior to the onset of inspiration, one of three may be seen:
1) Expiratory flow has not ceased
2) Positive pressure is measured with an esophageal balloon
3) Positive pressure is measured during an airway occlusion maneuver

❍ **Under what circumstances should dead space be added to the ventilator circuit?**

None.

❍ **What position is preferred for patients suspected of having an air embolism?**

Left lateral decubitus/Trendelenburg position.

❍ **What is the primary cause of hypercapnia?**

Hypoventilation.

❍ **A 50 year-old woman presents with pneumonia in the right lower and middle lobes. On 50% oxygen by facemask, her PaO_2 is 75 mmHg. Should the patient be positioned right side down or up?**

From an oxygenation perspective, right side up. Blood flow is gravity dependent. If the patient is positioned right side down, blood flow will preferentially go to the right side. However, because of the pneumonia, this will increase the amount of shunt, lowering the PaO_2 further.

From a pulmonary hygiene perspective, right side down. The infected material may move with gravity from the infected lung to the uninfected lung.

❍ **What is the treatment for carbon monoxide poisoning?**

100% oxygen, which increases carbon monoxide clearance by competing for binding to hemoglobin. Hyperbaric oxygen (oxygen provided at higher than atmospheric pressure) is recommended in more severe cases.

❍ **T/F: A normal $PaCO_2$ in a patient with an asthma exacerbation is a good sign.**

Maybe. A normal $PaCO_2$ in an asthmatic is good if the patient is feeling improved and less dyspneic. However, it can be a sign of impending respiratory failure if the patient continues to feel dyspneic and is working hard to breathe.

〇   **T/F: Oxygen should never be given to a hypoxemic patient with COPD who has chronic CO_2 retention.**

False. Oxygen should always be given to a patient who is hypoxemic.

〇   **What considerations should be addressed while giving the above patient oxygen?**

It has been shown that giving oxygen to a chronic CO_2 retainer usually does not result in a significant decrease in minute ventilation. The $PaCO_2$ will go up, but the rise is probably a result of changes in the ventilation-perfusion inequalities.

Oxygen should be given judiciously with repeat $PaCO_2$ determinations to ensure that the $PaCO_2$ does not rise precipitously.

〇   **What are the indications for chronic oxygen therapy?**

1. Resting $PaO_2 < 55$ mmHg or $SaO_2 < 88\%$.
2. Resting PaO_2 56-59 mmHg or SaO_2 89% in the presence of evidence of cor pulmonale or polycythemia.
3. During exercise if the PaO_2 falls below 55 mmHg or the SaO_2 below 88% with a low level of exertion.

〇   **What are the major mechanisms of hypoventilation and what clinical conditions are associated with each?**

1. Failure of the central nervous system ventilatory centers - drugs (narcotics, barbiturates) and stroke.
2. Failure of the chest bellows - chest wall diseases (kyphoscoliosis), neuromuscular diseases (amyotrophic lateral sclerosis) and diaphragm weakness.
3. Obstruction of the airways – asthma and chronic obstructive pulmonary disease.

〇   **How can hypoxemia secondary to hypoventilation alone be distinguished from other causes of hypoxemia?**

If the hypoxemia is from hypoventilation alone, the A-a O_2 gradient is normal. It is elevated in all other causes.

〇   **Changes in temperature, $PaCO_2$ or pH or the level of 2,3-diphosphoglycerate (2,3-DPG) cause a shift in the oxyhemoglobin dissociation curve. To cause a rightward shift, what are the changes that must occur?**

Increased temperature, increased $PaCO_2$, decreased pH and increased 2,3-DPG level. An easy way to remember this is that these conditions are often associated with decreased tissue oxygen levels. By right-shifting the curve, more oxygen is released from hemoglobin to the tissues.

〇   **How does the shape of the oxyhemoglobin dissociation curve effect the oxygen content of blood?**

Since SaO_2 does not increase significantly if the $PaO_2 > 60$ mmHg, the oxygen content of blood will increase significantly above this level only by increasing the hemoglobin concentration.

〇   **What are some common causes of respiratory alkalosis?**

Respiratory alkalosis is defined as a pH above 7.45 and a pCO_2 less than 35. Common causes of respiratory alkalosis include any process that may induce hyperventilation: shock, sepsis, trauma, asthma, PE, anemia, hepatic failure, heat stroke, exhaustion, emotion, salicylate poisoning, hypoxemia, pregnancy and inadequate mechanical ventilation.

○   **Calculate the alveolar-arterial oxygen (A-a O_2) gradient given the following arterial blood gas obtained at sea level: pH 7.24, $PaCO_2$ 60 and PaO_2 45.**

30 mmHg.

To calculate the alveolar-arterial oxygen gradient, you must first calculate the expected alveolar partial pressure of oxygen (PAO_2) using the alveolar gas equation. The alveolar gas equation is commonly written: $PAO_2 = PIO_2 - PaCO_2/R$, where PIO_2 is the partial pressure of oxygen in the inspired gas and R is the respiratory exchange ratio, commonly estimated at 0.8. PIO_2 is calculated as follows: $PIO_2 = FIO_2 (P_B - P_{H2O})$ where FIO_2 is the inspired concentration of oxygen (0.21 at sea level), P_B is the atmospheric pressure (760 mmHg at sea level) and P_{H2O} is the partial pressure of water (47 mmHg). At sea level, PIO_2 is equal to 150 mmHg. For this example, $PAO_2 = 150 - 60/0.8$ or 75 mmHg.

The A-a O_2 gradient is $PAO_2 - PaO_2$. Therefore, in this example, the A-a O_2 gradient is 75 - 45 or 30 mmHg.

○   **What is the normal A-a O_2 gradient?**

10 mmHg in a 20 year old.

○   **What are the principal mechanisms that lead to hypoxemia?**

Hypoventilation, diffusion limitation, shunt, ventilation-perfusion inequality, low inspired oxygen concentration, and low mixed venous oxygen in the presence of V/Q mismatch.

○   **Which of the above mechanisms is the most common?**

Ventilation-perfusion inequality.

○   **Why does hypoventilation lead to hypoxemia?**

Hypoventilation results in an increase in $PaCO_2$, which in turn decreases the PAO_2 (see the alveolar gas equation above).

○   **What are the effects of carbon monoxide on hemoglobin?**

Carbon monoxide bound to hemoglobin, carboxyhemoglobin, impairs tissue oxygenation by two mechanisms:
1:   It decreases oxygen carrying capacity by decreasing the amount of hemoglobin available for oxygen
       binding.
2:   It shifts the oxyhemoglobin dissociation curve to the left.

○   **What are the common clinical signs and symptoms of acute hypoxia?**

1. Respiratory: tachypnea, dyspnea and cyanosis.
2. Cardiovascular: tachycardia, palpitations, arrhythmias and angina.
3. Central nervous system: headache, impaired judgment, inappropriate behavior, confusion and seizures.

○   **What is the normal tidal volume and minute ventilation in an average 70 kg subject?**

The normal tidal volume (V_T) is 500 to 600 ml and the normal minute ventilation (V_E) is 5 to 6 L/min.

○   **Why do most asthmatics present with a decreased PCO_2?**

First, the increased $PaCO_2$ associated with the increased dead space stimulates the central nervous system chemoreceptors to increase minute ventilation, which in turn decreases $PaCO_2$. Also, the associated hypoxemia and sensation of dyspnea causes the patient to hyperventilate, which lowers the $PaCO_2$.

○   **Why do asthmatics eventually have an increased $PaCO_2$ if untreated?**

As the asthma attack continues untreated, the work of breathing will continue to increase. Eventually, the diaphragm fatigues and the patient hypoventilates. The hypoventilation, in association with the increased dead space and increased CO_2 production, increases the $PaCO_2$.

○   **What is the normal $PaCO_2$ and does it vary with age?**

The normal $PaCO_2$ is 35 to 45 mmHg and does not vary with age.

○   **What is the normal expected change in pH if there is an acute change in the $PaCO_2$?**

The pH will increase or decrease 0.8 units for every 10 mmHg decrease or increase (respectively) in $PaCO_2$.

○   **In chronic respiratory acidosis or alkalosis, what is the expected change in pH?**

The pH will increase or decrease 0.3 units for every 10 mmHg decrease or increase (respectively) in $PaCO_2$.

○   **What is the expected change in serum bicarbonate in chronic respiratory acidosis or alkalosis?**

Bicarbonate increases by approximately 3 mEq/L for each 10 mmHg increase in $PaCO_2$ in chronic respiratory acidosis. Bicarbonate decreases by 4 to 5 mEq/L for each 10 mmHg decrease in $PaCO_2$ in chronic respiratory alkalosis.

○   **What are the consequences of hypercapnia?**

Acute hypercapnia has physiologic consequences due to the increased $PaCO_2$ and to the decreased pH.

Physiologic effects of the $PaCO_2$ increase include:
1. Increase in cerebral blood flow.
2. Confusion, headache ($PaCO_2 > 60$mmHg), obtundation and seizure ($PaCO_2 > 70$mmHg).
3. Depression of diaphragmatic contractility.

The primary consequences of the decreased pH are on the cardiovascular system with in decreased cardiac contractility, decreased fibrillation threshold and vasodilatation.

○   **What are the consequences of hypocapnia?**

Acute hypocapnia has physiologic consequences due to the decreased $PaCO_2$ and to the increased pH.

Physiologic effects of the $PaCO_2$ decrease include:

1. Decreases in cerebral blood flow (this reflex is used in the management of neurologic disorders with high intracranial pressures as a short-term measure to decrease the increased intracranial pressure).
2. Confusion, myoclonus, asterixis, loss of consciousness and seizures.

The primary consequences of the increased pH are again primarily on the cardiovascular system with increased cardiac contractility and vasodilatation.

O   **A 32 year old male presents to the emergency room obtunded. Examination is significant for a respiratory rate of 8 and pinpoint pupils. An arterial blood gas reveals pH 7.28, $PaCO_2$ 55 and PaO_2 60. What is the cause of the hypercapnia?**

Acute narcotic overdose leading to hypoventilation.

O   **A 45 year old obese male presents with dyspnea, peripheral edema, snoring and excessive daytime sleepiness. A room air arterial blood gas shows the pH is 7.34, $PaCO_2$ 60 mmHg, PaO_2 58 mmHg and the calculated HCO_3^- is 28 mEq/L. What is the acid-base disturbance?**

Chronic compensated respiratory acidosis. If this were acute, the pH would be 7.28 with a normal HCO_3^-.

O   **What are the maximal oxygen concentrations that can be achieved by nasal cannula and facemask?**

6 L/min. of nasal cannula oxygen can achieve an FIO_2 of ~44%. A simple facemask can achieve an FIO_2 of ~60%.

O   **What is a nonrebreather mask?**

A nonrebreather mask has a one-way valve between the mask and a reservoir bag, such that the patient can only inhale from the reservoir bag (which contains 100% oxygen) and exhale through separate valves on the side of the mask.

O   **What is a Venturi mask?**

An oxygen delivery device in which room air and 100% oxygen are mixed in a fixed ratio allowing for the delivery of an accurate FIO_2 up to 50%.

O   **Why is a Venturi mask clinically useful?**

The Venturi mask is mostly commonly used for patients with chronic CO_2 retention and acute hypoxemia, where precise titration of the FIO_2 is necessary to prevent a precipitous increase in the $PaCO_2$.

O   **What should treatment for malignant hyperthermia include?**

A change in the anesthetic agent to remove possible triggers, administration of dantrolene and the procedure should be terminated.

O   **T/F: Severe auto-PEEP may cause pulseless electrical activity.**

True.

SHOCK PEARLS

O   **What is Beck's triad for the diagnosis of cardiac tamponade?**

Hypotension, elevated central venous pressure and a quiet precordium on auscultation.

O   **What hemodynamic changes are associated with sepsis?**

Increased cardiac index, decreased systemic vascular resistance (early stage), increased systemic vascular resistance (late stage), normal to decreased cardiac filling pressures and normal or elevated mixed venous oxygen saturation (early stage).

O   **What are the mechanisms of obstructive shock?**

Impedance to filling (e.g., tamponade and restrictive cardiomyopathies) and impedance to outflow (e.g., valvular stenosis and pulmonary embolism).

O   **What is pulsus paradoxus?**

A greater than normal decrease in systolic arterial pressure with inspiration.

O   **What is the differential diagnosis for pulsus paradoxus?**

Cardiac tamponade, status asthmaticus, severe chronic obstructive lung disease, pulmonary embolus, constrictive pericarditis and tension pneumothorax.

O   **What is the most common clinical finding in cardiac tamponade?**

Tachypnea followed by pulsus paradoxus and tachycardia.

O   **What are the underlying pathogenetic mechanisms of cardiogenic shock?**

Loss of contractile muscle, valvular failure, dysrhythmias and myocardial rupture.

O   **Can preload and PCWP be used as synonyms?**

No. PCWP is determined by juxtaventricular pressures, ventricular compliance and left ventricular end diastolic volume (LVEDV). LVEDV and preload are synonyms.

O   **What major conditions are associated with distributive shock?**

Sepsis, anaphylaxis, neurogenic shock and adrenal insufficiency.

O   **What is the pathogenesis of anaphylactic shock?**

Anaphylactic shock is an extreme manifestation of an immediate hypersensitivity reaction. It occurs through the interaction of an inciting antigen with mast cells and basophil-bound IgE. These effector cells then release numerous mediators that produce the clinical findings.

○ **What are the effects of septic shock on cardiac function?**

There is transient dilatation of one or both ventricles, reduced contractility and low ejection fraction. These changes typically last several days and normalize after 7 to 10 days.

○ **What are the typical clinical findings that distinguish distributive shock from other types of shock?**

Warm, well-perfused skin, wide pulse pressure and reduced diastolic blood pressure.

○ **What degree of blood loss is required to induce hypotension?**

20 to 25% of the blood volume.

○ **What are the initial priorities during shock resuscitation?**

Hemodynamic stabilization and cause-specific correction of the systemic and regional circulatory failure.

○ **What are the metabolic goals of shock resuscitation?**

Correction of oxygen debt, anaerobic metabolism and tissue acidosis.

○ **What is the importance of the splanchnic circulation during shock and the post-shock phase?**

The splanchnic tissues are preferentially underperfused relative to their metabolic demands during shock. Left uncorrected, this underperfusion is associated with increased morbidity and mortality.

○ **What is the significance of blood lactate determination in shock patients?**

Mortality is directly related to the degree of lactic acidosis.

○ **What is the role of catecholamines in the resuscitation of shock?**

Inotropic or vasopressor support once effective intravascular volume has been restored.

○ **What are the major drawbacks of catecholamine use in shock?**

Catecholamines can increase myocardial and systemic oxygen demands, induce arrhythmias and cause excessive vasoconstriction, resulting in ischemia.

○ **T/F: Normalization of vital signs, such as blood pressure and heart rate indicate complete resuscitation of shock.**

False. Systemic vital signs do not reliably reflect the physiologic end-points of shock resuscitation.

○ **What is the most common cause of death of shock patients?**

Multiple organ failure (MOF).

O   **Which parameter obtained on routine vital signs usually indicates a hypodynamic state?**

A narrowed pulse pressure.

O   **What are the typical PA catheter measurements in early septic shock?**

High cardiac output (CO), low systemic vascular resistance (SVR) and low or normal pulmonary capillary wedge pressure (PCWP). In later stages, CO will drop and SVR may rise.

O   **What is the treatment of septic shock?**

Volume infusion. Once euvolemia is achieved, vasopressor agents for hypotension or inotropic agents for inadequate tissue delivery of oxygen should be considered.

O   **How is cardiogenic shock managed?**

Euvolemia first, then inotropic or vasopressor support.

O   **What are typical PA catheter measurements in neurogenic shock?**

High or low CO, low SVR and low PCWP.

O   **How is neurogenic shock managed?**

Volume infusion followed by vasopressors, if needed.

O   **What are the characteristics of dopamine?**

It is primarily a dopaminergic agonist at low doses, a (-1 agonist at moderate doses and an (-agonist at high doses.

O   **T/F: Colloid solutions are preferred for resuscitation.**

False.

O   **What parameters indicate successful resuscitation?**

Return of normal vital signs and signs of end organ perfusion (as urine output and clear mentation).

O   **What are the indications for central venous cannulation?**

As a conduit for PA catheters, lack of peripheral access, CVP monitoring and infusion of vasoactive medications or medications requiring high flow veins.

O   **What is the preferred site for central venous catheterization?**

Controversial. All three major sites (femoral, internal jugular and subclavian) have advantages and disadvantages that must be weighed.

O   **What are the most common immediate complications of central venous catheterization?**

Pneumothorax, hemothorax, arrhythmias, arterial puncture, air embolus and malposition.

O   **What are the common delayed complications from central venous catheterization?**

Infection, thrombus formation, erosion through the SVC or atrium and delayed pneumothorax.

O   **What catheter tip culture result is suggestive of catheter sepsis?**

Greater than 15 colonies of the same organism.

O   **A patient has the following pulmonary artery catheter readings: Cardiac index (CI) of 2.0 L/min., CVP of 2 mm Hg, pulmonary artery occlusion pressure (PAOP) of 7 mmHg and SVR of 1600 dyne/sec/cm^2. What is the most likely diagnosis and what is the appropriate therapy?**

The patient is hypovolemic and would benefit from fluid resuscitation.

O   **A patient's pulmonary artery catheter readings reveal a CVP of 12 mm Hg, PAOP of 18 mm Hg, CI of 1.7 L/min. and SVR of 1650 dyne/sec/cm^2. What is the most appropriate treatment?**

Inotropic support. However, this must be judiciously balanced against the side effect of increasing myocardial oxygen demand. Depending on the patient's condition, an intraaortic balloon pump may be preferred. Echocardiography is necessary to rule out a structural cause for the decrease in cardiac index.

O   **How is the optimal filling pressure determined for a patient in cardiogenic shock?**

By obtaining a bedside Starling curve and plotting PCWP against CO after repeated small volume boluses or diuresis.

O   **Why has bicarbonate use been de-emphasized?**

Because of its harmful effects, which include hyperosmolarity, alkalemia, hypernatremia, paradoxical CSF acidosis and increased CO_2 production.

O   **T/F: Vasodilators should be employed early in the management of hemorrhagic shock.**

False.

O   **What are the CNS symptoms of acute volume loss?**

Lethargy and apathy, progressing to coma.

O   **What is the best initial fluid management for a patient with hemorrhagic shock?**

Lactated Ringer's.

O   **What are the signs of volume overload?**

Distended veins, bounding pulse, functional murmurs, peripheral edema and basilar rales.

O   **What are the characteristics of Class II hemorrhagic shock?**

Loss of 15 to 30% of circulating blood volume, tachycardia and a decrease in the pulse pressure.

O   **Which fluids flow faster through IV lines?**

Crystalloid and colloids are faster than red cells

○   **T/F: Colloid solution is the preferred solution for resuscitation.**

False. In terms of volume required, resuscitation with a colloid solution requires less volume than with a crystalloid solution. However, crystalloid is less expensive and yields no difference in outcome.

○   **T/F: Blood products should be given as the initial resuscitation fluid for patients with presumed large blood loss.**

False. Non-blood containing fluids can be infused faster and therefore will more quickly support perfusion. Blood, usually in the form of packed red blood cells, should be given early in those patients with presumed large volume blood loss.

○   **What are the indications for invasive arterial monitoring?**

Need for constant pressure monitoring due to a hemodynamic instability, vasoactive medications and need for frequent arterial blood gas monitoring.

○   **What are the preferred and acceptable alternative sites for arterial lines?**

The radial artery is preferred due to a very high percentage of collateral flow to hand. Femoral and dorsalis pedis arteries are acceptable.

○   **T/F: Non-invasive arterial pressure measurements are more accurate than direct arterial measurements.**

False.

○   **What patient populations are most likely to be helped by the use of the PA catheter?**

Patients with myocardial infarction and shock and those with shock refractory to volume loading, perioperative management of patients undergoing cardiac or vascular surgery and multiple trauma patients.

○   **What complications are associated with PA catheter usage?**

All possible complications inherent in any central venous access, as well as pulmonary artery rupture, higher incidence of arrhythmias and knotting of the catheter.

○   **At what points during insertion and use of PA catheters should the balloon be inflated?**

The balloon should be inflated to full volume (to obliterate the tip and avoid vessel puncture) as soon as it is in the SVC. It should remain inflated during any forward movement of the catheter and should be deflated prior to any withdrawal. Once in place, the balloon should be inflated only to the minimum volume necessary to obtain a pulmonary capillary wedge pressure (PCWP).

○   **What are normal pressures measured by the PA catheter?**

SVC: 1 to 6
PA: 15 to 30 / 5 to 15
PCWP: 6 to 12

○   **What are we really trying to measure when we measure the wedge pressure?**

Left ventricular end diastolic volume (LVEDV), a measure of the preload on the ventricle.

○   **What assumptions are made in using PCWP as a substitute for LVEDV?**

Several, most importantly that a stable relationship exists between LVEDP and LVEDV. Also that the PCWP is equal to the left atrial (LA) pressure which is equal to the LVEDP.

○   **How does PA diastolic pressure compare to PCWP as a measure of left heart filling pressures?**

Under normal conditions, the PCWP is usually within a few mmHg of PA diastolic pressure. Conditions common to critical illness make the two more disparate.

○   **How does PEEP affect PA catheter measurements?**

PEEP will increase the measured PCWP.

○   **What is VO_2?**

VO_2 is the measure of oxygen consumption.

○   **What is a normal VO_2?**

120 to 160 mL/m^2/min.

○   **What causes changes in VO_2?**

VO_2 decreases in hypothermia and paralysis. It increases during muscular activity, hyperthermia, hyperthyroidism and states of inflammation.

○   **When is oxygen consumption dependent on oxygen delivery?**

On the low end of the consumption vs. delivery curve, oxygen utilization is supply dependent.

○   **What does the oxygen saturation of venous blood (SvO_2) tell us in relation to DO_2 and VO_2?**

SvO_2 is a quick way of getting some idea about the adequacy of DO_2 and VO_2. Assuming arterial oxygen saturation of 95 to 100%, the venous saturation should be >70 to 75%. Less than this indicates supply is suboptimal. In some conditions such as sepsis, SvO_2 will actually be higher than normal even with inadequate tissue oxygenation.

○   **What are typical PA catheter measurements in hypovolemic shock?**

Low cardiac output, high systemic vascular resistance (SVR), low PCWP.

○   **When should the PA catheter be removed?**

When the information obtained is no longer being used to make clinical decisions. Not all critically ill patients need them.

○   **Ideally, how does the pulmonary artery catheter aid patient management?**

The usual scenario for placement of the catheter is when one of the parameters is in doubt, most commonly fluid status with unstable hemodynamics. The numbers obtained by the PA catheter may help guide management of fluids, diuretics and inotropic agents.

○   **How does phenylephrine differ from norepinephrine?**

Phenylephrine is a pure alpha-1 agonist. It can be used to increase SVR and BP. Like norepinephrine it is associated with a reflex bradycardia. Norepinephrine has both alpha-1 and beta-1 effects.

○   **Compare nitroglycerin and sodium nitroprusside.**

Both are vasodilators. Nitroglycerin is a greater venous vasodilator than an arterial vasodilator. In contrast, nitroprusside is primarily an arterial vasodilator. Unlike nitroprusside which is used primarily to manage hypertension and hypertensive crisis, nitroglycerin is also used to treat angina and congestive heart failure. Prolonged use of nitroprusside may cause thiocyanate toxicity.

○   **Discuss amrinone and milrinone.**

Both are phosphodiesterase inhibitors which have a relative selectivity for phosphodiesterase III, the predominant cAMP-specific form in cardiac tissue. They have an inotropic as well as a vasodilator effect. A major drawback is the development of thrombocytopenia. Milrinone is at least as effective if not more potent than amrinone. Another benefit of milrinone is that its incidence of thrombocytopenia is much lower than amrinone.

○   **Name three limitations of pulmonary artery catheter readings.**

PA catheter readings can fluctuate during respiratory variations and should therefore be read at end expiration. High PEEP can falsely elevate PA readings, particularly PAWP. Heart rates exceeding 120 beats/minute can also falsely elevate pulmonary artery diastolic pressure readings. A pressure change should be greater than 4 mmHg is considered clinically significant.

○   **What is the hallmark hemodynamic finding of constrictive pericarditis?**

Early diastolic dip and late diastolic plateau in the right ventricular pressure curve ("square root sign").

○   **What should be the first intervention in a patient with blunt chest trauma who has engorged neck veins, distant heart sounds, decreased breath sounds and hypotension after unsuccessful attempts to stabilize the patient with aggressive fluid replacement?**

Needle decompression of the chest for possible tension pneumothorax. If the shock state persists, an emergent pericardiocentesis for cardiac tamponade should be performed.

○   **How much of the pulmonary vascular bed needs to be occluded to cause shock in the setting of PE?**

More than 60% in patients with no prior cardiopulmonary disease.

○   **What is the survival benefit of patients with massive PE in shock given thrombolytic therapy compared to heparin alone?**

Faster clot lysis and improvement of right ventricular pressures have clearly been shown with thrombolytic agents. No study has ever been designed to demonstrate a survival advantage with thrombolytic agents.

O   **What is the treatment for patients with massive PE and hypotension?**

Vasopressors, heparin and thrombolytic agents. Embolectomy is a consideration as well.

O   **What is the classical hemodynamic picture seen in cardiogenic shock?**

Low cardiac index, high systemic vascular resistance and high pulmonary capillary wedge pressure (PCWP). The PCWP may not be elevated in right ventricular infarction.

O   **How much left ventricular muscle needs to be involved in the setting of an acute myocardial infarction (MI) to cause cardiogenic shock?**

40% or more.

O   **What are the causes of cardiogenic shock in the setting of an acute MI?**

> 40% loss of left ventricular myocardium, ventricular wall rupture, septal rupture, left ventricular aneurysm and acute mitral regurgitation due to papillary muscle rupture/dysfunction.

O   **What is the suspected diagnosis if a patient's blood pressure drops significantly with administration of nitroglycerin in the setting of an acute MI?**

Inferior wall MI with right ventricular involvement.

O   **By how much does an intraaortic balloon pump (IAPB) increase cardiac output?**

10 to 20%.

O   **Why does an IABP increase cardiac output?**

An IABP decreases left ventricular afterload and increases coronary perfusion.

O   **What seems to be the main predictor of survival of patients with cardiogenic shock due to an acute MI?**

Successful myocardial reperfusion.

O   **What is the first line treatment of a patient in cardiogenic shock due to RV infarction?**

Aggressive volume replacement as the right ventricle is "volume sensitive." Treatment may need to be guided by pulmonary artery catheter measurements.

O   **Describe the typical hemodynamic profiles of distributive and hypovolemic shock.**

Distributive shock: normal or low pulmonary capillary wedge pressure (PCWP), low systemic vascular resistance (SVR) and increased cardiac output (CO). Hypovolemic shock: low PCWP, increased SVR and low CO.

O   **How should cardiac output (CO) values be interpreted during shock resuscitation?**

CO is the total systemic blood flow. Normal or high values do not exclude cardiac dysfunction and do not assure matching of systemic or regional metabolic demands. Thus, CO determinations should be interpreted in combination with other hemodynamic and metabolic indicators.

○   **What is a common electrolyte abnormality associated with transfusion of packed red blood cells?**

Hypocalcemia secondary to citrate toxicity. Citrate, when rapidly infused, binds ionized calcium and therefore decreases the calcium level. Hyperkalemia may also develop with rapid packed red blood cell transfusion, especially if the patient is in renal failure or if the blood products are old.

○   **What is the calculation for mean arterial pressure (MAP) based on systolic (SBP) and diastolic pressure (DBP)?**

MAP = DBP + 1/3(SBP - DBP).

○   **What are the two most important determinants of coronary perfusion pressure?**

The two most important determinants of coronary perfusion pressure are diastolic blood pressure and left ventricular end-diastolic pressure:

CPP = DBP - LVEDP.

○   **What are the determinants of stroke volume?**

Preload, contractility and afterload.

○   **How would you calculate systemic vascular resistance (SVR)?**

$$\frac{MAP - CVP}{CO} \times 80 \, [dyne \times sec/cm^5]$$

○   **How would you calculate pulmonary vascular resistance (PVR)?**

$$\frac{Mean\ PAP - PCWP}{CO} \times 80 \, [dyne \times sec/cm^5]$$

○   **What is afterload?**

Afterload is either ventricular wall tension during systole or arterial impedance to ejection. Wall tension is usually described as the pressure the ventricle must overcome to reduce cavity size.

○   **What is the baroreceptor reflex?**

Increase in blood pressure stimulates peripheral baroreceptors located at the bifurcation of the common carotid arteries and the aortic arch. These baroreceptors then send afferent signals to the brainstem circulatory centers via the glossopharyngeal and vagus nerves, allowing an increase in vagal tone and, consequently, vasodilatation and a decrease in heart rate.

○   **Which drug most commonly causes true allergic reactions?**

Penicillin, which accounts for approximately 90% of all true allergic reactions. 95% of fatal anaphylactic reactions are caused by penicillin. Parenterally administered penicillin is more than twice as likely to cause a fatal anaphylactic reaction than the orally administered type.

○   **What is the treatment of choice for patients in anaphylactic shock?**

Epinephrine, 0.3-0.5 mg intravenously. If there is no IV access, inject the medication into the venous plexus at the base of the tongue.

○   **What is the most common source of sepsis in the elderly?**

Respiratory > Urinary > Intra-abdominal.

○   **What is the primary physiological alteration that occurs with shock?**

Inadequate tissue perfusion.

○   **What is pulmonary capillary wedge pressure (PCWP) an indication of?**

Left ventricle end diastolic pressure.

○   **How are PCWP readings used in the treatment of patients?**

It is used as a guide for fluid management in the patient.

○   **What is cardiogenic shock?**

Cardiac output is decreased because of inadequate myocardial contractility leading to inadequate tissue perfusion.

○   **What nursing assessment is essential during the administration of dopamine?**

Close blood pressure monitoring.

○   **What age groups are at risk for septic shock due to infection?**

The very young and the elderly.

○   **What may hypotension indicate in a patient with an MI?**

Cardiogenic shock.

○   **Define cardiac output.**

The amount of blood ejected from the heart per minute. It is expressed as liters per minute.

○   **Define stroke volume.**

The volume of blood ejected from the heart during systole.

○   **What is the most common cause of septic shock?**

Gram negative bacteria such as E. coli, Klebsiella pneumonia, and pseudomonas.

○   **What are the signs and symptoms of toxic shock syndrome?**

Temperature greater than 102 degrees F, rash, systolic blood pressure less than 90 mm Hg, and desquamation of the palms and soles of the feet.

○ **What are the major hemodynamic changes associated with cardiogenic shock?**

Decreased left ventricular function and decreased cardiac output.

CARDIOVASCULAR PEARLS

○ **What is the significance of large pulmonary V waves on the pulmonary capillary wedge tracing?**

Abnormally large V waves, greater than 10 mmHg greater than the mean pulmonary wedge pressure, represent filling of the left atrium during systole against an abnormally large left atrial pressure. It is most commonly found in mitral regurgitation, but can also be seen in mitral stenosis, congestive left ventricular failure, ventricular septal defects, Eisenmenger's complex, and, in rare instances, severe aortic regurgitation.

○ **What is the arterial oxygen saturation in a normal human? Venous saturation?**

The arterial saturation in a normal human is 95%. The venous saturation in a normal human is around 75%, but differs slightly, depending on where you measure.

○ **What is the normal cardiac output in an adult human?**

Approximately 4-6 L/min, depending on numerous factors such as body size, metabolic rate, posture, age, body temperature, anxiety, environmental heat and humidity and a host of other factors.

○ **What is the most accepted method of expressing cardiac output?**

Cardiac index. Cardiac index is the cardiac output divided by the body surface area in square meters.

○ **A 71 year-old male is admitted with hypotension, tachypnea and tachycardia. His HR is 122, systemic, blood pressure is 83/48 and the respiratory rate is 28. A Swan-Ganz pulmonary artery catheter is inserted and the cardiac output is 9.3 L/min. The pulmonary capillary wedge pressure is 11 mmHg and the SVR is 550 dynes-sec-cm^{-5}. What is this hemodynamic picture consistent with?**

Distributive shock, secondary to sepsis.

○ **What is the diagnosis of a patient with the following hemodynamic profile on Swan-Ganz hemodynamic monitoring: cardiac output- 3.4 L/min, PCWP- 6 mmHg, SVR- 1990 dynes-sec-cm^{-5}?**

Hypovolemic shock.

○ **A 71 year-old gentleman presents to the hospital with increasing shortness of breath, orthopnea, PND, and palpitations. He has a long history of recurrent CHF. His physical exam reveals bibasilar rales and he is hypotensive with a BP of 70/40 mmHg. Right heart catherization reveals the following: cardiac output- 2.6 L/min, BSA 1.9 m^2, PCWP 34 mmHg, SVR 2100 dynes-sec-cm^{-5}, PA pressure of 65/36 mmHg, and a right atrial pressure of 37 mmHg. What is the diagnosis?**

Cardiogenic shock from left heart failure.

O   **In the above patient, what is the preferred drug of choice for this problem?**

Dobutamine. This will reduce SVR and PCWP and potentially increase cardiac output. However, it is doubtful this patient will survive, given the profound cardiac depression found in this patient.

O   **What are the negative effects of PEEP on cardiovascular function?**

PEEP may reduce cardiac output by reducing venous return, by increasing pulmonary vascular resistance, and by shifting the interventricular septum to the left, thus reducing the left ventricular end diastolic volume.

O   **What are three ways that "best" PEEP can be determined?**

Compliance, oxygenation, and cardiac output.

O   **What is the role of corticosteriods in ARDS?**

Several studies have failed to show any benefit for the use of steroids in ARDS. There is some evidence that there may be a danger in using steroids in ARDS associated with sepsis. There is some evidence to suggest that in certain cases, in the late phases of ARDS steroids may reduce the fibrosis associated with late ARDS.

O   **What interventions have been shown to reduce the mortality of ARDS?**

Although a great number of studies have been done to reduce the mortality of ARDS, to date the only strong evidence for reduced mortality is in the computerized protocol for management of ventilator support. Other studies on a variety of interventions in the inflammatory cascade including prostaglandins and steroids have failed to show benefit. There is recent interest in the use of prone positioning for patients with ARDS.

O   **What are the most common presenting findings in ARDS?**

Tachypnea and hypoxemia.

O   **What are the NIH criteria for the diagnosis of ARDS?**

PaO_2/FiO_2 ratio < 200, bilateral infiltrates, wedge pressure < 18.

O   **What is the cause of hypoxemia in ARDS?**

An increase in alveolar fluid causes reduced diffusion of oxygen into capillaries, thus increasing the shunt.

O   **What is the mortality of ARDS?**

Most series show a mortality of 40-60%. Some research protocols have shown a reduction to 25-30%.

O   **What are the most risk factors for ARDS?**

Sepsis, trauma, aspiration, multiple transfusions, shock, pulmonary contusions. However, many other systemic and local insults may trigger ARDS.

O   **Why is the pulmonary artery wedge pressure an important feature in the diagnosis of ARDS?**

The presence of a significantly elevated wedge pressure implies that the pulmonary edema may be hydrostatic and therefore due to left ventricular dysfunction rather than alveolar or pulmonary dysfunction and ARDS— that is, noncardiogenic pulmonary edema.

○ **Does PEEP improve ARDS?**

PEEP commonly improves oxygenation; however, it does not reduce the amount of total lung water, which is the marker for the amount of pulmonary edema present.

○ **What is the distribution of pulmonary edema in ARDS?**

Routine chest x-ray appears to show a diffuse distribution. However, CAT scan studies reveal an increased involvement in the dependent portions of the lung fields.

○ **What are the x-ray findings in ARDS?**

Diffuse ground-glass-like infiltrates that do not follow anatomical boundaries, usually bilateral.

○ **What complications are associated with ARDS?**

Barotrauma leading to pneumothorax, pulmonary infection, pulmonary hypertension, multisystem organ failure.

○ **What are the three phases of ARDS?**

Acute or exudative (up to 6 days), proliferative phase (4 to 10 days), chronic or fibrotic phase (after 7 days).

○ **What is the role of PEEP in ARDS?**

Maintain alveolar inflation and functional residual capacity.

○ **The most feared complication associated with Extra Corporeal Membrane Oxygenation?**

Intracranial hemorrhage.

○ **The risks and complications of pericardiocentesis include?**

Cardiac tamponade, myocardial infarction, intra-abdominal injuries and pneumothorax.

○ **Decompensated shock is characterized by?**

Hypotension and low cardiac output.

○ **In hypovolemia from hemorrhage, the blood pressure is maintained until?**

The blood volume falls by 25% to 30%.

○ **The indications for calcium therapy include?**

Documented or suspected hypocalcemia, hyperkalemia, hypermagnesemia, and calcium channel blocker overdose.

❍   **The treatment of choice for patients with supraventricular tachycardia and cardiovascular compromise?**

Adenosine, but in the event that vascular access is not available quickly synchronized cardioversion becomes the treatment of choice.

❍   **When should atropine be used for the treatment of bradycardia?**

Only after adequate ventilation and oxygenation have been established, since hypoxemia is a common cause of bradycardia.

❍   **T/F: Defibrillation is indicated for the treatment of asystole.**

False. Defibrillation is the definitive treatment for ventricular fibrillation or pulseless ventricular tachycardia. The treatment for asystole is epinephrine.

❍   **After a cardiac arrest, the most common reason for poor perfusion is?**

Cardiogenic shock resulting from arrest-associated myocardial ischemia.

❍   **What is the immediate treatment of choice in ventricular fibrillation?**

Immediate defibrillation, starting at 200 Joules. If unsuccessful, repeat at 300 Joules, and if still unsuccessful, repeat a third time at 360 Joules. If still unsuccessful, start CPR and achieve adequate ventillation with immediate intubation.

❍   **What is the treatment of choice for hemodynamically stable ventricular tachycardia?**

Intravenous bolus of lidocaine at 1 mg/kg, followed by an infusion of lidocaine at 2-4 mg/min. A repeat bolus should be given at .5 mg/kg, 15 minutes after the initial bolus.

❍   **In CPR, what is the ventilation to compression ratio for one rescuer?   For two rescuers?**

1 rescuer: 2 breaths to 15 compressions
2 rescuers: 1 breath to 5 compressions

❍   **Non-traumatic cardiac arrest patients are most likely to be successfully resuscitated from what abnormal rhythm?**

Ventricular fibrillation. Success is time dependent, generally declining at a rate of 2-10% per minute.

❍   **If a defibrillator is available, what is the immediate treatment of a patient with ventricular fibrillation?**

Unsynchronized countershock at 200J.

❍   **What is the differential diagnosis of pulseless electrical activity?**

Tension pneumothorax, acidosis, MI, PE, OD, cardiac tamponade, hypoxia, hypovolemia, hyperkalemia and hypothermia (TAMPOT plus 4H is the pnemonic).

❍   **What is the differential diagnosis of asystole?**

Drug overdose, acidosis, hyperkalemia, hypothermia, hypokalemia, hypoxia.

O   **How much myocardial damage from an acute myocardial infarction is necessary to result in congestive heart failure?**

Congestive heart failure is usually evident clinically if more than 25% of the left ventricle is infarcted.

O   **How much functional loss of left ventricular myocardium is required to result in cardiogenic shock?**

40%.

O   **What is the most common cause of death related to acute myocardial infarction?**

Ventricular fibrillation, occurring within the first hour following symptoms.

O   **What percentage of patients with acute myocardial infarction develop cardiogenic shock?**

10%.

O   **A 60 year-old patient suffers an acute inferior myocardial infarction. Three hours after he arrives in the hospital, he develops ventricular fibrillation and is successfully defibrillated back to normal sinus rhythm within 30 seconds. He makes a full recovery and has no further post-MI complications. What does his ventricular fibrillation episode indicate with regard to his subsequent risk of sudden death?**

This episode has no bearing on his subsequent risk of sudden death. Ventricular fibrillation in the immediate setting of an acute myocardial infarction has no prognostic significance.

O   **What arrhythmias that occur in patients with acute myocardial infarction require temporary pacing?**

Complete heart block (3° AV block); new LBBB; new bifasicular block; marked sinus bradycardia with ischemic pain, hypotension, CHF, frequent PVCs or syncope despite atropine; and Mobitz II type 2° AV block.

O   **A 54 year old gentleman admitted two days ago with an acute anterolateral myocardial infarction suddenly develops atrial fibrillation with a ventricular rate of 135/min. He subsquently complains of substernal chest discomfort. His BP is 135/70. What is the most appropriate immediate action to be taken?**

Synchronized DC cardioversion.

O   **T/F: The presence of occasional PVCs is a reliable predictor of ventricular fibrillation following acute myocardial infarction.**

False.

O   **A 58 year-old gentleman is admitted with an acute anteroseptal myocardial infarction. He is in pulmonary edema clinically, confirmed by CXR. His blood pressure is 122/76, his HR is 122. Despite two doses of 80 mg of intravenous furosemide, he remains in pulmonary edema. A Swan-Ganz pulmonary artery catheter is inserted and his initial hemodynamics reveal a cardiac output of**

3.1 L/min and a pulmonary capillary wedge pressure of 27 mmHg. What is the most appropriate pharmacologic agent in this setting?

Intravenous Dobutamine, at a dose of 5 to 20 mcg/kg/min.

○ **What is the current recommended therapy for patients with large anterior myocardial infarctions?**

Reperfusion therapy with thrombolytics, beta-blockers, intravenous nitroglycerin and ACE inhibitors to limit and retard ventricular remodeling. Intravenous heparin in a sufficient dose to prolong the APTT to 1.5 to 2.0 times control should be started on admission and continued to discharge. In patients with large akinetic apical segments or mural thrombi, oral anticoagulation with warfarin is indicated for 3-6 months.

○ **What is the significance of pericarditis following acute myocardial infarction?**

Pericarditis occurs in about 20% of patients with acute myocardial infarction, more likely in Q wave infarcts than non-Q wave infarcts. Patients with pericarditis usually have significantly larger infarcts, lower ejection fractions and a higher incidence of congestive heart failure. The presence of pericarditis and/or pericardial effusion following acute myocardial infarction is associated with a higher mortality.

○ **A previously healthy 65 year-old man is admitted with an acute inferior myocardial infarction. Within several hours, he is hypotensive (BP 90/60) and oliguric. Insertion of a pulmonary artery catheter reveals the following pressures: pulmonary artery wedge pressure, 3 mmHg, pulmonary artery, 21/3 mmHg and mean right atrial pressure, 11 mmHg. What is the best treatment for this man?**

Fluids, until his wedge pressure is between 16-20 mmHg.

○ **What two groups of patients are more likely to present with "silent" myocardial infarction?**

Patients with diabetes mellitus and the elderly.

○ **What is the most useful test for the immediate confirmation of the diagnosis of acute myocardial infarction?**

The electrocardiogram. It is diagnostic of acute myocardial infarction in about two-thirds of patients.

○ **What is the usual time sequence of the onset, peak and duration of the elevation of CK-MB levels in an acute myocardial infarction?**

CK-MB levels are usually elevated within 4-6 hours following the onset of acute myocardial infarction, peak at approximately 18-24 hours and usually return to normal at 36-48 hours following an uncomplicated infarction.

○ **At what time frame do LDH levels peak following acute myocardial infarction?**

24-48 hours.

○ **What are the absolute contraindications to intravenous thrombolytic therapy?**

Major surgery, organ biopsy or major trauma within 2 weeks; significant GI or GU bleeding within 2 months; known or suspected aortic dissection; known or suspected pericarditis; known intracranial tumor; previous neurosurgery or hemorrhagic cerebrovascular accident at any time; acute severe hypertension

(>200 mmHg systolic or >120 mmHg diastolic; head trauma within one month; thrombotic cerebrovascular accident within two months and active internal bleeding, excluding menses.

❍   **What are the relative contraindications to intravenous thrombolytic therapy?**

Mild to moderate hypertension (>180 mmHg systolic and/or >110 mmHg diastolic); cardiopulmonary resuscitation for < 10 minutes; puncture of non-compressible vessel; recent TIAs; thrombotic cerebrovascular accident between 2 to 6 months ago; diabetic retinopathy; active peptic ulcer; known bleeding diathesis or current anticoagulant usage; pregnancy; and exposure to streptokinase or APSAC within the last 6-9 months (does not apply to prospective t-PA administration).

❍   **Which age group has the greatest reduction in mortality following the administration of thrombolytic therapy in the presence of an acute myocardial infarction?**

Patients over the age of 65, and more specifically, those patients over age 75.

❍   **What are the two most common and serious side effects of streptokinase and APSAC?**

Hypotension and hypersensitivity reaction, which is antigen mediated and manifested by vomiting, itching and swelling.

❍   **What is the rationale for intravenous heparin administration being started concommitantly with t-PA administration?**

Because the plasma clearance time of t-PA is 4-8 minutes, the coronary rethrombosis rate in the absence of intravenous heparin is significantly increased and ranges between 20-30%. With concommitant heparin administration and continued heparinization for at least 24 hours following t-PA therapy, the coronary rethrombosis rate is reduced to approximately 5-10%.

❍   **What is the preferred agent of choice in the treatment of atrial fibrillation occurring in the setting of acute myocardial infarction?**

Beta-blockers. Alternative agents, such as procainamide or amiodarone, are particularly useful in converting atrial fibrillation to sinus rhythm.

❍   **What is the percentage of rupture of the free wall of the left ventricle occurring in patients who die as a result of acute myocardial infarction?**

10%. This event occurs between 1 and 5 days following infarction and is almost always fatal.

❍   **Should anticoagulation be routinely administered to patients with acute myocardial infarction?**

For large anterior myocardial infarctions, it is currently recommended to administer intravenous heparin, until discharge, in a dose sufficient to prolong the APPT to 1.5 to 2 times normal. Those patients with a mural thrombus or a large akinetic apical segment should be treated with warfarin for three to six months. Long-term anticoagulation is generally indicated in patients with a dilated, severely hypokinetic left ventricle.

❍   **Pericarditis occurs in what percentage of patients with acute myocardial infarction?**

10-20%, as defined by the presence of a friction rub.

O   **What is the significance of infarct-related pericarditis?**

Patients with infarct-related pericarditis usually have larger infarcts, have lower post-MI ejection fractions, and a higher incidence of congestive heart failure and serious ventricular arrhythmias. Patients with infarct-related pericarditis and/or the presence of pericardial effusion have a higher mortality, again related to infarct size.

O   **What is the most important prognostic determinant following acute myocardial infarction?**

Infarct size.

O   **Are thrombolytic agents effective in non-Q wave MI?**

No, there is no evidence to support their use. In fact, some published data suggest that their use may be detrimental.

O   **What is the prognosis of patients presenting with Q wave MI complicated by acute mitral regurgitation?**

Prognosis is quite compromised with an approximate one-year survival of only 50%.

O   **What are the major precipitants of AMI?**

In over half of patients with AMI, no precipitantant can be indentified. However, some precipitatory factors which have been identified include emotional stress, surgical procedures, neurological disturbances and perhaps extreme physical excertion. Circadian changes in plasma catecholamines and cortisol may also play a precipitatory role.

O   **What is the most common presenting symptoms of AMI?**

Chest pain. Unlike aortic dissectioin, this pain often waxes and wanes, and over time will become severe. It usually lasts greater than 30 minutes and is frequently described as crushing, constricting, or as pressure. The pain is typically retrosternal and frequently radiates to the jaw and the ulnar aspect of the left arm. In some patients, particularly the elderly, AMI may present as a sumptoms of actue left ventricular failure rather than chest pain.

O   **What are the other typical symptoms of AMI?**

Diaphoresis, apprehension, sense of doom, nausea and vomiting, which occur in greater than 50% of patients with transmural infarction. These latter symptoms, and perhaps the others to some extent, occur presumably due to the Dezold-Jarisch reflex. Nausea and vomiting occur more frequently in inferior myocardial infarction.

O   **What are the most common atypical presentations of AMI?**

Congestive heart failure, angina without a prolonged or severe episode and atypical pain location.

O   **What is a silent AMI?**

Population studies suggest that 20 to 60% of non-fatal MIs are unrecognized by the patient and are found on subsequent routine ECG. About one-half of these MIs are truly silent with no identifiable symptoms recalled by the patient. Unrecognized or silent infarction occurs more often in patients without previous anginal syndromes and is more common in diabetics and hypertensive patients.

O What are the most common physical findings in AMI?

There really aren't any, and findings depend upon the absence or presence of actue complications such as congestive heart failure, acute mitral regurgitation or cardiogenic shock. Most patients will appear to be in some distress. Of note, a <u>fourth heart sound</u> is almost universally present in ptients with acute MI.

O Describe the chactaresistic pattern of creatine phospkokinase (CK-MB) elevation in AMI.

CK exceeds normal levels in 4 to 8 hours after onset of MI. The <u>mean</u> peak for CK is 24 hours, but can range from 8 to 58 hours. Peak levels occur earlier in patients who receive reperfusion therapy, with <u>mean</u> peak CK rise occurring at approximately 12 hours. In gnereal, CK levels normalize 3 to 4 days after onset of pain.

O What are the main causes of false positive CK evelation?

Muscle disease, alcohol intoxication, diabetes mellitus, skeletal muscle trauma, vigorous exercise, convulsion, PE and thoracic outlet syndrome.

O Desribe the characteristics pattern of lactate dehydrogenase (LDH) elevation after onset of AMI.

Levels exceed normal by 24 to 48 hours after AMI onset, peak 3 to 6 days after onset and normalize 8 to 14 days after onset. Total LDH, while sensitive, is not specific. Fractionation into its isoforms increases specificity, since myocardium contains primarily LDH-1, where other sources contain primarily the other LDH isoforms. Thus, an LDH-1 to LDH-2 ratio of greater than 1.0 is a commonly used cutoff for diagnosing recent MI. Use of LDH analysis should be limited to those patients with normal CK measurements.

O What other serum markers are important in diagnosing AMI?

Recently, it has been shown that the Troponins demonstrate high concordance with CK-MB, and they apper a bit earlier in the course of MI. Also, subsets of the Troponins are highly specific for myocardial damage. Lastly, recent published data suggest that the amount of Troponia released may be an independent marker of survival.

O What factors contribute to defining patients at high risk for complications from thrombolytic therapy? (This is <u>not</u> the same as contraindications).

Advanced age, systollic blood pressure greater than 200 and/or diastolic blood pressure greater than 110 that is not effectively lowered with medical therapy in the emergency depaprtment, history of definite stroke and recent surgery. There are many other factors which add incremental risk, such as CHF, hypotension and anterior locations, to name a few. It should be noted that high risk patients receive the greatest benefits from thrombolytic therapy.

O Routine use of oxygen is or is not beneficial in acute MI?

The rationale is that hypoxemia is bad for myocardial necrosis and that ventilation perfusion mismatch is common in patients with acute MI, particularly after heparin administration. However, the routine use of oxygen in non-hyproxemic patients has not been proven beneficial. Regardless, most centers recommended routine use of oxygen per 6 to 12 hours to ensure adequate oxygenation of the patient.

O What are the major contraindications to beta-blocker therapy in AMI?

All patients with AMI should be considered for beta-blocker therapy, and only patients with a major contra-indication should be excluded. These contraindications include pulmonary edema with rales greater than one-third of the lung fields, marked hypotension, PR-interval greater than 24 seconds or advanced hear block, bradycardia (heart rate less than 55-60 bpm) or known bronchospasm (active or history of severebronchospasm). Several studies have repeatedly shown that beta-blocker therapy reduces mortality and recurrent ischemia when administered early in acute myocardial infarction.

○   **What are the indications for temporary transvenous pacing in AMI?**

Temporary pacing is indicated in patients at high risk with developing complete heart block, particularly new bifascicular bundle branch block or LBBB. Patients who develop a systole, Mobitz type II and complete heart block will may also benefit from temporary transvenous pacing. It should be noted, however, that the use of temporary pacing has never been statistically proven to improve prognosis.

○   **What is the most common sustained supraventricular arrhythmia in AMI?**

Sinus tachycardia. About one-third of patients will develop sinus tachycardia in the first days after acute AMI. The most common causes are anxiety, persistent pain, and left ventricular failure.

○   **What is the least common sustained supraventricular arrhythmia AMI?**

Atrial flutter, occurring in 1-3%.

○   **What is the most common sustained arrhythmia in AMI?**

Probably ventricular fibrillation, occurring in up to 10% of patients, and is seen more commonly in transmural infarction. The majority (60%) of VF events in AMI patients occur within 4 to 6 hours, and 80% by 12 hours. This "Primary" VF have been thought not to affect prognonis when treated rapidly, but some investigators have suggested this may indicate a worse prognosis.

○   **What is the best treatment for accelerated idioventricular rhythm (AIVR)?**

AIVR, characterized by a wide QRS rhythm with a rate faster than the atrial rate and less than 150 bpm, should not be treated, unless associated with a very significant drop in blood pressure. This rhythm is seen frequently in the early stages of AMI and occurs more often in patients with early reperfusion. However, it is neither sensitive nor specific enough to be considered a reliable marker for reperfusion.

○   **What is reperfusion injury?**

The acceleration of myocardial cell necrosis after reperfusion. It is characterized by rapid cellular swelling and wide spread architectural disruption. It is likely the acceleration of necrosis occurs in cells already destined to die, but it is possible that reperfusion may cause necrosis of reversably injured myocardial cells as well.

○   **What factors predict development of pericarditis in AMI patients?**

Pericarditis usually occurs 1 day to 6 weeks after AMI. It is more common in males, Q wave infarction and patients with congestive heart failure. Some reports suggest that pericarditis occurs in 10 to 20% of patients, but pericardial effusion without evidence of pericarditis is far more common.

○   **How common is acute myocardial infarction (AMI)?**

It is estimated that one and a half million myocardial infarctions occur every year in the U.S. Approximately one third of the patients with these events will die, with one half of deaths occurring prior to institution of medical therapy.

O   **What is the pathophysiology of acute MI?**

In general, acute occlusion secondary to thrombosis is considered the most common cause of AMI. Most transmural MIs are associated with complete obstruction whereas non-transmural MIs may be done to thrombosis alone, spasm with associated thrombosis, or, in significantly obstructed arteries, may be done to hypoxemia or hypotension.

O   **What is the most common cause of acute coronary thrombosis?**

Plaque disruption. Not all plaques have the same propensity to rupture. Characteristics rendering plaques "vulnerable" to disruption include: high lipid content, thin (as opposed to thick) fibrous cap, monocyte content and shear forces present.

O   **What is the mortality benefit from aspirin alone in acute myocardial infarction with thrombolytic therapy and in subsequent reinfarction?**

Aspirin reduced mortality from acute myocardial infarction by 23% and reduced non-fatal reinfarction by 49%. When used with thrombolytic therapy, there was a 40-50% reduction in mortality from acute myocardial infarction.

O   **A 63 year-old gentleman presents to the ICU with moderate substernal chest pressure and lightheadedness for 90 minutes. His BP on admission is 80/40 and his HR is 110/min and regular. Physical exam reveals JVD to the angle of the jaw, a right parasternal S3 gallop, an apical S4 gallop and clear lungs on auscultation. ECG reveals 2 mm ST elevation in leads II, III, and aVF with reciprocal ST depression in V1-V3. What is the most likely diagnosis and what is the most appropriate initial therapy?**

Inferior myocardial infarction with right ventricular infarction. Following 160-325 mg of aspirin administration, thrombolytic therapy and a large bolus of intravenous saline followed by a moderately high infusion rate of saline are indicated. If the patient remains hypotensive despite adequate intravenous saline, as measured by the development of lung congestion on auscultation, intravenous Dobutamine is indicated.

O   **A 70 year-old man is admitted to the hospital with chest pain of 3 hours duration. ECG demonstrates anterior ST elevation for which he is given aspirin, r-TPA, heparin and intravenous nitroglycerin. His symptoms resolve. Serum chemistries reveal a peak CPK of 1800 and a CK-MB fraction of 15%. He is eventually transferred out of the CCU and his hospitalization is uneventful until day 5, when he develops sudden, severe shortness of breath. BP is 110/75 and his pulse is 125 and regular. Examination reveals a new systolic murmur. What would the most appropriate therapeutic intervention be?**

Intravenous sodium nitroprusside. This patient is most likely suffering from rupture of the left ventricular septum and subsequent defect, a not uncommon complication of MI. Afterload reduction is key to stabilization until surgical repair of the VSD can be performed, usually in about 8-12 weeks, after the infarct has healed. If nitroprusside fails to stabilize the patient, intra-aortic balloon counterpulsation and intravenous nitroglycerin should be employed.

O   **What are the major complications of left ventricular aneurysms?**

LV thrombus formation (with the subsequent risk of thromboembolic events), CHF and ventricular arrhythmias.

O   **What is unstable angina (UA)?**

In the presence of ECG or enzyme evidence of AMI, the term UA is usually applied in three historical circumstances: 1) New onset angina of Canadian class III or worse; 2) Angina at rest as well as with minimal exertion; 3) More severe or prolonged angina in the context of a previous stable pain pattern. The more traditional definitions require one or more of these historical features with electrocordiographic changes, but many centers will classify patients as having unstable angina in the absence of ECG cardio findings.

O   **How does one treat unstable angina?**

UA, like AMI, is usually due to plaque rupture followed by platelet aggregation and thrombosis. Thus, the use of aspirin, heparin, or both is essential. Of note, while aspirin and heparin are both effective, there has not been definitive proof that one is better than the other, or that the combination is better than either agent alone. Use of nitroglycerin, beta-blockers and calcium channel blockers are also standard therapy.

O   **What is the definition of unstable angina?**

Unstable angina is an intermediate coronary syndrome between angina pectoris and acute myocardial infarction. Its presence depends on one or more of the following three historical features: 1) crescendo angina (more severe, prolonged or frequent) superimposed on a pre-existing pattern or relatively stable, exertion-related angina pectoris, 2) angina pectoris of new onset (within one month) which is brought on by minimal exertion or 3) angina pectoris at rest as well as minimal exertion. Variant angina, which is also characterized by angina at rest, has sometimes been considered to be a form of unstable angina, but it is pathogenitically different from unstable angina.

O   **What is the classification of unstable angina?**

Class I: New onset, severe or accelerated angina occurring within two months of presentation without rest pain. Also included in this class are patients whose angina is more frequent, severe, longer in duration or precipitated by substantially less exertion than previously.

Class II   Patients with angina at rest during the preceding two months but not within the last 48 hours.

Class III   Patients with rest angina at least once within the preceding 48 hours.

O   **What are some of the clinical circumstances in which unstable angina occurs?**

Secondary unstable angina refers to patients, usually with underlying obstructive CAD, in whom the imbalance between myocardial oxygen supply and demand causing the instability results from conditions that are extrinsic to the coronary vascular bed. This includes patients who have anemia or hypoxemia that cause reduced myocardial oxygen supply, as well as patients with fever, infection, aortic stenosis, uncontrolled hypertension, thyrotoxicosis, extreme emotional upset and tachyarrhythmias that cause increased myocardial oxygen demand.

Primary unstable angina, the most common form of unstable angina, occurs in the absence of an identifiable extracoronary condition and in patients who have not suffered an acute myocardial infarction within the preceding two weeks. Post-infarction unstable angina is present in patients who develop unstable angina within two weeks of a documented acute myocardial infarction; it occurs in approximately 20% of patients following infarction.

O   **What is the etiology of primary unstable angina?**

Atherosclerotic plaque rupture followed by platelet aggregation and thrombus formation. Aggregation of platelets and thrombus formation, usually superimposed on an atherosclerotic plaque, obstructs blood flow to the affected myocardium sufficiently long enough to cause ischemia and clinical symptoms, but not long enough to result in myocardial necrosis and infarction, as recanalization of the affected coronary artery occurs, usually within 20 minutes to one hour after the onset of plaque rupture. Unstable angina is often a precursor of acute myocardial infarction, and the two conditions share a common pathophysiologic link.

O   **What factors portend a worse prognosis and signify a high-risk patient in those with unstable angina?**

Older patients, patients with continued rest pain despite medical therapy, and patients with thrombi, complex coronary morphology or multivessel disease on coronary angiography. Patients who have ischemia detected on ambulatory electrocardiographic monitoring and those with significant ST-T wave abnormalities at presentation are also at higher risk and tend to have an unfavorable outcome.

O   **What is the most useful diagnostic test in the evaluation of patients with unstable angina?**

Coronary angiography.

O   **What is the hallmark of drug therapy for patients admitted with unstable angina?**

Intravenous low molecular-weight heparin and at least 81 mg of aspirin daily. Intravenous nitroglycerin is strongly recommended for patients with Class II or Class III unstable angina, but one must keep in mind to increase the dose of intravenous heparin during intravenous nitroglycerin administration as nitroglycerin reduces the efficacy of heparin.

O   **What is the role of thrombolytic therapy in unstable angina?**

None. To date, no clinical trial has shown any benefit of thrombolytic therapy, presumably because thrombi in unstable angina tend to be platelet-rich, not fibrin-rich, and thus resistant to thrombolytic therapy.

O   **What are some other highly efficacious drug therapies in patients with unstable angina?**

Beta-blockers have been shown to be highly effective in reducing the frequency and duration of both symptomatic and silent myocardial ischemic episodes. Calcium channel antagonists, while not as efficacious as beta-blockers in reducing myocardial oxygen demand, are highly effective in reducing symptoms and ischemic episodes, but should not be used as monotherapy. In fact, monotherapy with nifedipine in unstable angina is associated with an increase in non-fatal myocardial infarctions within the first 48 hours after initiation of therapy.

O   **Rales are present on exam in a 50 year-old man with recent anterior wall MI. What can you say about the pulmonary artery occlusion ("wedge") pressure?**

It is likely above 20 to 25 mmHg.

O   **What is preload?**

The wall stress that the ventricle (LV) sees at the end of diastole, which is determined by venous return. In the normal heart, when preload increases, the LV distends, the resting length of the sarcomere increases and the LV can generate greater pressures more rapidly, augmenting stroke volume.

O   **What is afterload?**

The load against which the LV must contract as systole begins—that is, the pressure the LV must generate to open the aortic valve and then eject blood.

○   **You evaluate an elderly female with hypotension. During the assessment, the patient complains of chest pain. She is diaphoretic; her lips are dusky; her radial pulse is faint and slow. Jugular venous distension is present, but the lung fields are clear. Glancing at her bedside monitor, you conclude that her central venous line has migrated distally, since there is a right ventricular pressure tracing. What's going on?**

The patient is having a right ventricular infarction with hypotension secondary to *right* ventricular failure. The physical exam findings are classic. The central line has not migrated, but is showing a characteristic "ventricularized" tracing.

○   **Sustained ventricular tachycardia is well controlled in a 55 year-old man post non-Q wave MI with lidocaine 2 mcg/mL. He has a known history of ischemic cardiomyopathy. Day 3 of his admission, his speech becomes slurred, he is lethargic, and, when aroused, becomes very agitated. What should you do?**

Inform the doctor that this patient has classic findings of lidocaine toxicity, and you should strongly consider stopping this drug. Elderly patients and patients with heart failure of hepatic insufficiency are especially at risk.

○   **A 72 year-old woman admitted to the ICU with pulmonary edema is much improved after overnight diuresis. Soon after you note that she is 4L negative in fluid balance, she develops polymorphic VT requiring cardioversion. Her regular medications include 80 mg bid of furosemide. What is a likely etiology?**

Beware of electrolyte abnormalities, especially hypokalemia, inducing torsades pointes in CHF patients after vigorous diuresis – especially in patients on chronic diuretics.

○   **A 65 year-old man with known severe hypertension, past CHF and COPD is intubated for acute pulmonary edema and suspected pneumonia. BP is 190/110; 92 saturation is 94% on 60% O_2. You successfully lower his blood pressure to 140/80 with intravenous sodium nitroprusside. However, the patient develops chest pressure and you note that his O_2 saturation is now 86%. What happened?**

Two effects of nitroprusside are likely culprits. Non selective dilation of the pulmonary arteriolar bed can worsen ventilation-perfusion mismatch, especially in patients with COPD or pneumonia, and cause desaturation. "Coronary steal" (reduced perfusion to coronary arteries with fixed obstruction in the setting of arteriolar dilation by nitroprusside) may lead to ischemia and chest pain.

○   **Despite appropriate medical therapy, including combination diuretics, a 75 year-old woman with reduced systolic function in acute pulmonary edema remains oliguric. What "mechanical" intervention may increase her urine output?**

Intubation or CPAP, if she can tolerate it. A large portion of her (already decreased) cardiac output is going to her overworked diaphragm. Decreasing her work of breathing will allow better perfusion of her kidneys, and can lead to dramatic diuresis.

○   **The above patient has a 2.5L diuresis after intubation. She is placed on a CMV mode with 10 of PEEP. The next morning, her lungs are clear. You attempt a T-piece wean, but note rales throughout both lung fields within minutes. What are three possible explanations?**

1) You've increased her work of breathing prematurely (i.e., before maximizing other therapies). 2) Coronary artery disease with concomitant ischemia may be contributing. 3) You've abruptly withdrawn potent cardiopulmonary effects of positive pressure ventilation. By increasing intrathoracic pressure, CMV and PEEP decrease the pressure gradient for venous blood flow from the great vessels to the right atrium, thereby decreasing preload; positive pressure against the heart can also have afterload-reducing effects.

○ **What are two reasons why dobutamine, in general, is a superior inotrope in heart failure to dopamine?**

Dobutamine acts as a peripheral dilator and reduces systemic vascular resistance, whereas dopamine, even at intermediate infusion rates, may cause peripheral vasoconstriction. Tachycardia and arrhythmias tend to occur more frequently with dopamine than dobutamine.

○ **What are the most common causes of atrial fibrillation?**

Hypertension with hypertensive heart disease is very common. Ischemic heart disease, mitral or aortic valvular heart disease, cor pulmonale, dilated cardiomyopathy, hypertrophic cardiomyopathy (particularly the obstructive type), alcohol intoxication ("holiday heart syndrome"), hypo- or hyperthyroidism, pulmonary embolism, sepsis, hypoxia, pre-excitation syndrome and pericarditis are also common causes.

○ **What are the common causes of SVT?**

Myocardial ischemia, myocardial infarction, congestive heart failure, pericarditis, rheumatic heart disease, mitral valve prolapse, pre-excitation syndromes, COPD, ethanol intoxication, hypoxia, pneumonia, sepsis and digoxin toxicity.

○ **What is the treatment of paroxysmal SVT?**

In a hemodynamically stable patient, intravenous adenosine. If unsuccessful, then intravenous verapamil, beta-blockers or procainamide. In the unstable patient with hypotension, angina or heart failure, immediate synchronized cardiversion should be performed.

○ **What is the most common supraventricular arrhythmia in the perioperative setting?**

Atrial fibrillation.

○ **What is the key feature of Mobitz Type I 2° AV block (Wenkebach)?**

A progressive prolongation of the PR interval until the atrial impulse is no longer conducted through to the ventricle, resulting in a dropped QRS. Almost always transient, atropine and transcutaneous/transvenous pacing is required for the rare instances of symptoms or cardiac instability.

○ **What is the feature of Mobitz II 2° AV block?**

A constant PR interval until one sinus beat fails to conduct through to the ventricule, resulting in a dropped QRS. Since this rhythm is indicative of His bundle damage, and 85% of patients with this rhythm eventually develop complete heart block, temporary followed by permanent pacing is usually required.

○ **What is the most common cause of Mobitz Type II 2° AV block?**

Coronary artery disease with acute myocardial ischemia. In the absence of coronary artery disease, the most common cause is degenerative AV node and His bundle disease.

○   **What is the appropriate management of the above arrhythmia in a patient on no SA or AV nodal suppressant drugs?**

Temporary transvenous pacemaker insertion followed by permanent pacemaker implantation.

○   **What is the treatment of Torsades de Pointes?**

Torsades de Pointes is a polymorphic form of ventricular tachycardia that occurs in the setting of long repolarization. Treatment usually requires removal of the reversible triggers that caused Q-T prolongation, such as hypokalemia and drugs, such as quinidine and other antiarrhythmic agents, pacing the atrium or ventricle to increase cardiac rate and rapidly infusing magnesium sulfate.

○   **Which antiarrhythmic agents increase defibrillation threshold (i.e., increase the energy requirement for successful defibrillation)?**

Lidocaine, mexiletine, encainide, flecainide, propafenone, amiodarone and verapamil.

○   **What are the most common initial rhythms in adults with cardiac arrest?**

VF and VT.

○   **For VF or unstable VT, what is the most important intervention to optimize chances for successful resuscitation?**

Defibrillation.

○   **What is the primary indication for atropine?**

Symptomatic bradycardia.

○   **A 28 year-old presents with hemodynamically stable paroxysmal supraventricular tachycardia (PSVT) at a rate of 170. What is the drug of choice?**

Vagal maneuvers are tried first. If unsuccessful, adenosine is the drug of choice.

○   **What is the treatment of choice for rapid atrial fibrillation in a patient with Wolff-Parkinson-White syndrome?**

Cardioversion if the patient is unstable, otherwise procainamide (20 to 30 mg/min up to 17 mg/kg) is the treatment of choice. The infusion should be stopped if further widening of the QRS or hypotension occurs.

○   **Tachycardia occurs after a cardiac arrest and is treated successfully with defibrillation and epinephrine. Should this post-resuscitation rhythm be treated?**

If the patient has a pulse and is hemodynamically stable, no treatment may be necessary. If epinephrine is responsible for the tachycardia, it should resolve quickly. Sustained sinus tachycardia should not be allowed to persist, however, as it increases myocardial oxygen consumption.

○   **What physical findings suggest an acute aortic dissection?**

BP differences between arms and/or legs, cardiac tamponade, and aortic insufficiency murmur.

❍ **What type of abnormal cardiac rhythm can be slowed through Valsalva maneuvers and/or carotid massage?**

Supraventricular rhythms.

❍ **Name some common Valsalva maneuvers.**

Holding the breath, stimulation of the gag reflex, ipecac, squatting, pressure on the eyeball, or immersing the face in ice.

❍ **What are some of the adverse effects of lidocaine?**

Drowsiness, nausea, vertigo, confusion, ataxia, tinnitus, muscle twitching, respiratory depression, and psychosis.

❍ **80–90% of patients who experience sudden non-traumatic cardiac arrest are in what rhythm?**

Ventricular Fibrillation. Early defibrillation is the key. In an acute MI, the infarction zone becomes electrically unstable. Ventricular fibrillation is most common during original coronary occlusion or when the coronaries begin to reperfuse.

❍ **When administering CPR, what is the ventilation to compression ratio for one rescuer?**

2 breaths to 15 compressions.

❍ **What is the ventilation to compression ratio for two rescuers?**

1 breath to 5 compressions.

❍ **What is the most common side effect of β-blockers?**

Fatigue, which occurs early in treatment; and depression, which occurs later.

❍ **What is the most common cause of death within the first few hours following an MI?**

Cardiac dysrhythmias, generally V-fib.

❍ **What are the ECG findings on a patient with hypokalemia?**

Flattened T-waves, depressed ST segments, prominent P-waves, prominent U-waves, and prolonged QT and PR intervals.

❍ **What are the ECG findings on a patient with hyperkalemia?**

Peaked T-waves, prolonged QT and PR intervals, diminished P-waves, depressed T-waves, QRS widening, levels exceeding 10 mEq/L, and a classic sine wave.

❍ **What is the first ECG finding for a patient with hyperkalemia?**

The development of tall-peaked T-waves at levels of 5.6–6.0 mEq/L, which are best seen in the precordial leads.

○   **What are the causes of hyperkalemia?**

Acidosis, tissue necrosis, hemolysis, blood transfusions, GI bleed, renal failure, Addison's disease, primary hypoaldosteronism, excess po K+ intake, RTA IV, and medications such as succinylcholine, b-blockers, captopril (Capoten), spironolactone, triamterene, amiloride, and high dose penicillin.

○   **What is the first-line of treatment for ventricular fibrillation in a hypothermic patient?**

Bretylium, NOT lidocaine.

○   **In the elderly, what is a common side effect of verapamil?**

Constipation.

○   **Name some drugs that when overdosed can lead to cardiac arrhythmias and death.**

Digoxin, antiarrhythmic drugs, cocaine, tricyclic antidepressants, darvon/darvocet, and phenothiazines.

○   **What does Beck's Triad signify?**

Acute pericardial tamponade.

○   **What metabolic conditions will potentiate the toxic cardiac effects of digoxin?**

Hypokalemia and hypercalcemia.

○   **What effect does morphine have on preload and afterload?**

Morphine decreases both preload and afterload.

○   **Does furosemide affect preload or afterload?**

Furosemide decreases preload.

○   **What should you be aware of when taking vital signs in a patient with an arteriovenous fistula?**

Do not take the blood pressure in the arm containing the fistula.

○   **During the first hours after a myocardial infarction, why is it important to monitor the patient's ECG?**

Arrhythmias are the leading cause of death following an infarct.

○   **What is the most common antiarrhythmic agent used for the treatment of PVCs.**

Lidocaine.

○   **The presence of more than 6 PVCs per minute puts the patient at risk for what arrhythmia?**

Ventricular tachycardia leading to ventricular fibrillation.

O   **A client is admitted to the ICU with a decreased level of consciousness, a BP of 45/15, shallow respirations, and ventricular tachycardia on the monitor. What should you do first?**

Prepare to defibrillate the patient and call for help in resuscitation.

O   **After a patient is brought back to a normal sinus rhythm following defibrillation, what medication will most likely be ordered?**

IV lidocaine bolus and an infusion begun.

O   **An MD orders streptokinase for treatment of an MI. What is the most harmful complication of this medication that you should assess for?**

Bleeding.

O   **Following a femoropopliteal bypass, you frequently assess pulse, skin color, temperature, and pain on the affected side. What is the rationale?**

A high priority should be placed on detecting the patency of the graft. Any symptoms of occlusion should be reported immediately.

O   **A patient complains stating that when he takes his sublingual nitroglycerin, he gets a burning sensation under his tongue. What is your response?**

This is normal. If this sensation does not occur, then the medication is stale.

O   **What cardiac abnormality can occur with theophylline levels above 35 mcg/ml?**

Ventricular arrhythmias.

O   **Describe some the commons signs of cardiogenic shock.**

Low blood pressure, oliguria, crackles in the lungs, rapid and weak pulse, and diminished blood flow to the brain.

O   **What is the rationale for giving morphine sulfate to a client in acute congestive heart failure?**

It helps to alleviate the anxiety caused by pulmonary edema and hypoxia.

O   **Following heart surgery, it is contraindicated to place the patient's legs in a flexed position, or to place anything behind their knees while lying supine. Explain the rationale?**

It may cause pooling of blood in the lower extremities, thus decreasing circulation.

O   **Following heart surgery, your client experiences persistent bleeding from the incision site. What drug will the physician most likely order to help stop this bleeding?**

Protamine sulfate.

O   **What important side effect of Inderal (propranolol hydrochloride) should you assess for?**

Slowed pulse rate and associated dyshythmias.

○   **You instruct your client to never stop Inderal abruptly. Why?**

Rebound hypertension may occur.

○   **What is the correct compression rate for 2 man CPR in an adult?**

80-100 per minute.

○   **What is the best position for a patient in acute CHF, and why?**

High Fowler's. It decreases venous return and allows for maximum lung expansion.

○   **What are some of the toxic effects of lidocaine?**

Confusion, dizziness, tremors, blurred vision, tinnitus, numbness and tingling of the extremities, hypotension, convulsions, and coma.

○   **What is the mechanism of action of lidocaine upon heart tissue?**

It decreases automaticity of the His-purkinje fibers and raises the stimulation threshold in the ventricles.

○   **What is the cause of pain in a myocardial infarction?**

Oxygen deprived ischemic cardiac muscle.

○   **During mitral valve stenosis, blood is unable to fully empty into the left ventricle thereby causing back up of blood from the left atrium into what vessel?**

The pulmonary vein.

○   **What information does an EKG provide?**

It reflects the electrical impulses transmitted through the heart and can be an indicator of the functional status of the heart muscle and contractile responses of the ventricles.

○   **What is the main goal of therapy for a patient in congestive heart failure?**

Increase cardiac output.

○   **What is the purpose of a cardiac catheterization?**

To assess the extent of coronary artery blockage.

○   **How can percutaneous transluminal coronary angioplasty cause a fluid volume deficit?**

The contrast medium used can act as an osmotic diuretic and diuresis can result.

○   **What is the most common cause of death following a myocardial infarction?**

Cardiac dysrhythmias.

○   **What is cardiogenic shock?**

Cardiac output is decreased because of inadequate myocardial contractility leading to inadequate tissue perfusion.

○ **Following CPR, a patient regains consciousness. What emotional state is he likely to be in?**

Confusion, anxiety, and disorientation. You should offer emotional support and orient the patient as best as possible.

○ **In the absence of renal or cardiac problems, what should be the normal urine output in a patient who is adequately hydrated?**

30-35 ml/hour or greater.

○ **What vital sign should be monitored closely during administration of nitroglycerin?**

Blood pressure.

○ **What should be done if premature ventricular contractions (PVCs) at a rate of 8-10 per minute are noticed on a patient's monitor?**

Notify the physician. PVCs greater that 5-6 per minute are considered dangerous.

○ **What wave is usually indistinguishable on the EKG when atrial fibrillation is present?**

The "P" wave.

○ **How could a patient's pulse be described if atrial fibrillation is present?**

Irregular with a variable rate.

○ **In a patient taking Quinidine, Lasix, and Digoxin, what is a potential side effect of combining these medications?**

Digoxin toxicity. Lasix can cause hypokalemia leading to toxicity, and Quinidine can cause elevated serum Digoxin levels.

○ **What would be a priority nursing diagnosis following an MI?**

Impaired Gas Exchange because of the poor oxygenation and dysrhythmias that can occur following an MI.

○ **What would be the purpose of administering digoxin intravenously to a patient with CHF?**

Lanoxin can help strengthen myocardial contractions and thus help increase cardiac output, which will help reduce pulmonary edema.

○ **What type of drug is enalapril maleate (Vasotec), and how does it work?**

It is an angiotensin-converting enzyme (ACE) inhibitor that decreases the level of angiotensin II. This will then decrease peripheral vascular resistance and blood pressure is lowered.

○ **Why is there a potential for blood clot formation in a patient with atrial fibrillation?**

The ineffective contractions of the atria cause blood stasis and thus clot formation.

○   **What is the primary effect of nitroglycerin?**

Peripheral vasodilatation which reduces myocardial oxygen consumption and workload.

○   **What is the reason for administering epinephrine to a patient during CPR?**

It stimulates the adrenergic receptors of the heart and can increase impulse conduction, thus stimulating some cardiac activity.

○   **What should be a primary nursing assessment during the administration of TPA?**

Signs and symptoms of spontaneous bleeding.

○   **Why should a patient who has just had an MI avoid the Valsalva maneuver?**

It can cause a change in heart rate, arrhythmias, increased intrathoracic pressure, and blood clot dislodgment.

○   **What are the common side effects of nitroglycerin?**

Headache, hypotension, and dizziness.

○   **What is coronary percutaneous transluminal coronary angioplasty (PTCA)?**

A balloon tipped catheter is inserted into the coronary artery and compresses the plaque in hopes of dilating the artery.

○   **When chest pain occurs, what is the time interval for administration of nitroglycerin tablets?**

Immediate administration with subsequent does at 5 minute intervals until the pain has resolved or a total of three tablets have been taken.

○   **At what time is a patient at greatest risk of dying from a myocardial infarction?**

The first 24-48 hours after an acute myocardial infarction.

○   **For a patient in cardiac arrest, what is the first priority?**

Establish an airway.

○   **What is the drug of choice for reducing premature ventricular contractions?**

Lidocaine hydrochloride.

○   **What is the breath to compression ratio when administering two person CPR?**

1 breath for every 5 compressions.

○   **What may hypotension indicate in a patient with an MI?**

Cardiogenic shock.

○ **How does nitroglycerine help relieve the pain associated with angina and an MI?**

It causes coronary artery vasodilatation leading to an increase in blood flow to cardiac muscle.

○ **Define cardiac output.**

The amount of blood ejected from the heart per minute. It is expressed as liters per minute.

○ **What are the characteristics of angina pectoris?**

Substernal pain that lasts 2-3 minutes, and may radiate to the neck, shoulders, or jaw. It is usually described as vise-like or constricting pain. It may be associated with diaphoresis, nausea, and a feeling of impending doom.

○ **What is indicated by anginal pain that persists for more than 20 minutes and is not relieved by nitroglycerine?**

A developing myocardial infarction.

○ **What is considered a normal central venous pressure?**

2-3 mm Hg (or 3-15 cm of water).

○ **Why is CVP monitored?**

To assess the need for fluid replacement, estimate blood volume deficits, and evaluate circulatory pressure in the right atrium.

○ **What are the major hemodynamic changes associated with cardiogenic shock?**

Decreased left ventricular function and decreased cardiac output.

○ **What does the term "silent myocardial infarction" indicate?**

An MI that produces no symptoms.

○ **What does a CPK-MB level greater than 5% of the total CPK indicate?**

An acute myocardial infarction.

○ **What are the findings in cardiogenic shock?**

Tachycardia, cyanosis, weak pulse rate, diaphoresis, pale cool skin, blood pressure below 80 mm Hg, and oliguria of less than 30 ml of urine per hour.

○ **What is the chest compression rate for adult CPR?**

80-100 times per minute.

○ **What are the major complications of an acute myocardial infarction?**

Thromboembolism, cardiogenic shock, left ventricular rupture, acute heart failure, and arrhythmias.

○   **What is the treatment of choice for patients with pulseless ventricular tachycardia?**

Defibrillation.

TRAUMA PEARLS

○ **Following blunt trauma to the chest, what type of injury is implied by the presence of pneumomediastinum, subcutaneous emphysema and a large air leak following tube thoracostomy?**

Tracheobronchial tear or disruption.

○ **What is a flail chest?**

When a segment of the thoracic cage becomes anatomically and functionally separated from the rest of the cage. It is caused by double fractures of 3 or more contiguous ribs, most often due to blunt trauma. The flail segment moves inward when the rest of the chest moves outward. This results in ineffective ventilation.

○ **What is the major cause of hypoxemia in patients with flail chest?**

Pulmonary contusion.

○ **How is flail chest treated?**

Analgesics and ventilatory support when respiratory failure occurs. The use of stabilizing devices is controversial.

○ **A patient presents after receiving a blow to the forehead. Her neck is hyperextended and she complains of weakness in her arms and minimal weakness in her lower extremities. What is the most likely diagnosis?**

Central cord syndrome.

○ **What is the most common cause of shock in patients with blunt chest trauma?**

Pelvic or extremity fracture.

○ **What organ is most commonly injured in blunt trauma?**

The spleen. Generalized abdominal pain with radiation to the left shoulder subsequent to blunt trauma suggests splenic rupture. Splenic rupture can also occur following minor trauma in a patient with infectious mononucleosis.

○ **What is a defect in the chest wall into which air is pulled during inspiration called?**

Sucking chest wound.

○ **How big does a chest wall defect have to be to redirect the incoming air away from the trachea?**

If the wound is > two-thirds the diameter of the trachea it will become the path of least resistance and become a sucking chest wound, making effective spontaneous ventilation impossible.

○   **What is the usual mechanism by which traumatic diaphragmatic hernias occur?**

Penetrating wounds to the lower chest and upper abdomen cause the majority of diaphragmatic hernias. Children are more likely to suffer this injury from blunt trauma.

○   **Define increased intracranial pressure.**

ICP > 15 mmHg.

○   **What valve is most commonly injured with blunt trauma?**

Aortic valve.

○   **What is the most likely cause of a new systolic murmur and ECG infarct pattern observed in a patient with chest trauma?**

Ventricular septal defect.

○   **What are the features of anterior cord syndrome?**

Loss of anterior cord function, which involves complete motor paralysis and loss of pain and temperature sensation. Posterior column function, which includes light touch, vibration and proprioception, is preserved.

○   **What are the features of central cord syndrome?**

There is a loss of motor function worse in the upper extremities than the lower extremities. The perianal area is often spared. Cervical hyperextension is the usual mechanism.

○   **What are the features of the Brown-Sequard syndrome?**

Caused by penetrating injury to one side of the spinal cord, it presents with an ipsilateral motor deficit and contralateral loss of pain and temperature sensation. Light touch is usually absent on the side of the lesion.

○   **Which pattern of partial cord injury has the worst rate of functional recovery?**

Anterior cord syndrome.

○   **What is the most common type of incomplete spinal cord injury?**

Central cord syndrome.

○   **A radial pulse on exam indicates a BP of at least _____.**

80 mmHg.

○   **A femoral pulse on exam indicates a BP of at least_____.**

70 mm Hg.

○   **A carotid pulse indicates a BP of at least_____.**

60 mm Hg.

O   **A trauma patient presents with decreasing level of consciousness and an enlarging right pupil. What is the most likely diagnosis?**

Uncal herniation with oculomotor nerve compression.

O   **Name the clinical signs of basilar skull fracture.**

Periorbital ecchymosis (raccoon's eyes), retroauricular ecchymosis (Battle's sign), otorrhea or rhinorrhea, hemotympanum, bloody ear discharge, hearing loss and anosmia.

O   **A trauma patient presents with anisocoria, neurological deterioration or lateralizing motor findings. What is the treatment?**

Hyperventilation, mannitol IV and phenytoin.

O   **A trauma patient presents with subcutaneous emphysema. What is the diagnosis?**

Pneumothorax or pneumomediastinum. If subcutaneous emphysema is severe, consider major bronchial injury.

O   **What rib fracture has the worst prognosis?**

First rib. First and second rib fractures are associated with bronchial tears, vascular injury and myocardial contusions.

O   **What is the basic disorder contributing to the pathophysiology of compartment syndrome?**

Increased pressure within closed tissue spaces compromising blood flow to muscle and nerve tissue.

O   **What are the two basic mechanisms for elevated compartment pressure?**

1) External compression: by burn eschar, circumferential casts, dressings or pneumatic pressure garments. 2) Volume increase within the compartment: hemorrhage into the compartment, IV infiltration or edema due to post-ischemic swelling.

O   **Which two fractures are most commonly associated with compartment syndrome?**

Tibial (anterior compartment involvement) and supracondylar humeral fractures.

O   **What signs & symptoms would be noted for a compartment syndrome involving the superficial posterior compartment of the leg?**

Pain on active and passive foot dorsi-flexion and plantar-flexion and hypesthesia of the lateral aspect of the foot (sural nerve).

O   **Where is the most common site of compartment syndrome?**

Anterior compartment of the leg, which contains the tibialis anteriorus, extensor digitorum longus, extensor hallucis longus and peroneus muscles, as well as the anterior tibial artery and deep peroneal nerve.

O   **What is the dose of methylprednisolone used to treat acute spinal cord injury?**

30 mg/kg load over 15 min in the first hour followed by 5.4 mg/kg per hour over the next 23 hour.

O   **What is the sensory innervation to the nipple, umbilicus and perianal region?**

Nipple   - T5.
Umbilicus - T10.
Perianal - S2-4.

O   **Describe the key features of spinal shock.**

Hypotension with bradycardia.

O   **Bacterial endocarditis secondary to soft tissue infections may be caused by which two organisms?**

Staphylococcus aureus and *Staphylococcus epidermidis*.

O   **What factors increase the likelihood of wound infection?**

Dirty or contaminated wounds, stellate or crushing wounds, wounds longer than 5 cm, wounds older than 6 hours and infection prone anatomic sites.

O   **In general, what is the maximum time limit for salvaging an ischemic limb?**

Six hours. Less if all the arterial collaterals are injured as well.

O   **What are the treatment modalities used to minimize the risk of infection in an open fracture?**

Antibiotic therapy, aggressive surgical debridement, fracture stabilization and meticulous wound care.

O   **What are typical clinical findings of a compartment syndrome?**

Tenseness of the involved compartment to palpation, pain with passive motion, paresis and intact distal pulses. Loss of distal pulses is a late sign.

O   **What clinical findings are suggestive of arterial injury after penetrating trauma?**

Physical findings such as a cold limb, absent or diminished pulse, difference in extremity systolic pressures or the presence of a bruit or thrill may indicate an arterial injury. Some arterial injuries are best treated in the operating room without the delay of an arteriogram, especially when there is threatened viability of the limb.

O   **What is fat embolism syndrome?**

A clinical syndrome characterized by respiratory insufficiency, mental status changes and thrombocytopenia with petechiae. Fat emboli arise primarily from the marrow of fractured long bones. The pulmonary findings are essentially indistinguishable from that of adult respiratory distress syndrome (ARDS).

O   **T/F: Any penetrating trauma from the nipple line to the inguinal ligament can produce an intra-abdominal injury.**

True. Due to the upward movement of the diaphragm during normal respiration to the level of the fifth intercostal space, any penetrating injury below this can cause an abdominal injury.

○   **What injuries are most commonly missed by CT scan?**

Hollow viscus, pancreas and diaphragm.

○   **What is the most commonly injured organ following penetrating trauma to the abdomen?**

The liver followed by the small bowel.

○   **What type of trauma, penetrating or blunt, places the stomach at greatest risk for injury?**

Penetrating trauma carries a far greater risk to the stomach with a reported incidence of injury of 12% versus 1% for blunt trauma.

○   **T/F: Blood in the NG tube is a sensitive sign for gastric injury during penetrating trauma.**

False. Blood per NG tube is only present in a third of patients with penetrating injury to the stomach.

○   **T/F: Serum amylase is a useful marker for ruling out pancreatic injury.**

False. Amylasemia is neither sensitive nor specific for pancreatic injury.

○   **With all types of abdominal injury, what is the organ most often injured?**

Liver.

○   **What is the most common indication for exploratory laparotomy following blunt trauma?**

Splenic injury.

○   **What are the clinical manifestations of abdominal compartment syndrome?**

<u>Respiratory</u>: decreased compliance, increased airway pressures, increased pulmonary vascular resistance, hypercarbia and hypoxemia.
<u>Cardiovascular</u>: decreased cardiac output.
<u>Abdomen</u>: decreased splanchnic flow.
<u>Renal</u>: oliguria.

○   **What formula should be used to calculate fluid requirements for resuscitation of a burn victim?**

4 ml/kg / %TBSA / day.
One-half of this is given in the first 8 hours.

○   **What number of points is the best verbal response worth in the Glasgow coma scale?**

5.

○   **What number of points is the best motor response worth in the Glasgow coma scale?**

6.

O   **A patient opens his eyes to voice, makes incomprehensible sounds and withdraws to painful stimulus. What is his GCS?**

9.
Glasgow coma scale:

Eye opening	Best verbal response	Best motor response
4 spontaneously	5 oriented x 3	6 obeys command
3 on request	4 confused conversation	5 localizes pain stimulus
2 to pain	3 inappropriate words	4 flexes either arm appropriately
1 no opening	2 incomprehensible sounds	3 flexion withdrawal
	1 no response	2 extension withdrawal
		1 no response

O   **A patient has sustained blunt trauma to the chest that results in pneumothorax. Multiple chest tubes have not controlled the air leak. What complication should you suspect?**

A Bronchial tear. Bronchoscopy is necessary for diagnosis, followed by emergency thoracotomy.

O   **Can tetanus occur after surgical procedures?**

Yes. While most cases of tetanus in the US occur after minor trauma, there have been numerous reports of tetanus following general surgical procedures, especially those involving the GI tract.

O   **What is the required dose of Ringer's solution in a 16 year old with 20% body surface burn?**

4 liters in the first 8 hours (500 ml per hour). The patient should receive 250 ml/hour over the next 16 hours. The Parkland formula = (4 ml)(kg body weight)(% burned). Give 1/2 the volume in the first 8 hours and the other half in the next 16 hours. Management after this should be judged clinically. Urine output should be maintained at 50 ml/hr in adults and 0.5 to 1 ml/kg/hour in children.

O   **You help stabilize a multiple trauma victim whose injuries include mild head injury, scalp lacerations and a femur fracture. The next morning you note a new right hemiparesis and confusion. Furthermore his oxygen saturation has dropped to the low 90s and his urine output is declining. The patient is noted to have petechiae on his chest and in his conjunctivae. What is the most likely diagnosis?**

Fat embolism.

O   **What complications are associated with hypothermia?**

Coagulopathy, confusion, disorientation, decreased immune response, platelet dysfunction, reduced cardiac function, decreased cardiac output, vasoconstriction and hypotension.

O   **What measures can be instituted to treat hypothermia?**

Increasing the room temperature, using intravenous fluid and blood warmers, heating ventilator gases and using warming blankets.

○   **As the patient re-warms, what problems can arise?**

Development of metabolic acidosis, shivering, hypotension and tachycardia.

○   **List the four mechanisms of heat loss from the body.**

The four mechanisms of heat loss are:

1) Radiation: Transfer of heat from a warm to a cold body via electromagnetic radiation.
2) Convection: Air abutting the body is heated by way of its direct contact to the patient. Since warm air is less dense it rises and is replaced by cooler air.
3) Evaporation: Water on the body's surface evaporates, the latent heat of vaporization comes from the patient whose temperature consequently falls.
4) Conduction: This is the direct transfer of heat energy through a substance.

○   **Which are the sites that contribute to evaporative heat loss?**

Evaporation accounts for heat loss from the skin and respiratory tract.

○   **What complications can result from heat stroke?**

Renal failure, rhabdomyolysis, DIC and seizures. Remember antipyretics will not help.

HEAD AND NECK PEARLS

O **What is the most feared complication of an infection in the retropharyngeal space?**

Mediastinitis.

O **What fascial space is involved in Ludwig's angina?**

The submandibular space.

O **What is the most common origin of infection in patients with Ludwig's angina?**

Dental abscesses.

O **What are the most common local findings in patients with Ludwig's angina?**

Swelling of the floor of the mouth and tongue.

O **What is the most common cause of death in Ludwig's angina?**

Asphyxiation.

O **What is the most common indication for surgical drainage in patients with Ludwig's angina?**

Failure of antibiotic therapy.

O **What are the most important organisms in Ludwig's angina?**

Oral anaerobes.

O **A patient presents with well-demarcated swelling of the lips and tongue. She was started on an antihypertensive agent three weeks ago. What is the most likely agent?**

Angiotensin-converting enzyme inhibitor. Although angioneurotic edema may occur anytime during therapy, it is most likely to occur within in first month when using and ACE inhibitor.

O **What are the two major risk factors for ocular candidiasis?**

Indwelling venous catheters and intravenous drug abuse.

PULMONARY PEARLS

O   **How long may hypoxemia last beyond upper abdominal or thoracic surgery?**

Hypoxemia may last days to weeks after thoracic or upper abdominal surgery. This correlates with a reduced FRC and an increased closing capacity.

O   **What is IPPB?**

Intermittent positive pressure breathing. Early studies showed its application reduced the incidence of complications over controls. However, it is no more effective than deep breathing exercises and incentive spirometry. IPPB is best reserved for those patients where active lung inflation is not possible even with patient cooperation (such as muscular dystrophy and kyphoscoliosis).

O   **What is non-invasive mechanical ventilation?**

It is the application of positive pressure breathing via the use of a tight fitting mask. The mask can be uncomfortable. The advantage may be in that often obviates the need for intubation and the risks thereof.

O   **What is CPAP?**

Continuous positive airway pressure.

O   **What is BiPAP?**

Bilevel positive airway pressure.   An expiratory pressure and an inspiratory pressure are dialed in per the needs of the patient. A tightly fitting nasal mask the interface to the patient.

O   **What is the cause of hypoxemia in ARDS?**

An increase in alveolar fluid that causes a reduction in the diffusion of oxygen into the capillaries, increasing the shunt.

O   **What are the major risk factors for ARDS?**

Sepsis, trauma, aspiration, multiple transfusions, shock and pulmonary contusions. Many other systemic and local insults may trigger ARDS.

O   **Why is the pulmonary artery wedge pressure an important feature in the diagnosis of ARDS?**

The presence of a significantly elevated wedge pressure implies that the pulmonary edema is due to left ventricular dysfunction rather than alveolar dysfunction.

O   **Does PEEP improve ARDS?**

PEEP commonly improves oxygenation. However, it does not reduce the amount of total lung water.

O   **What complications are associated with ARDS?**

Pneumothorax, pulmonary infection, pulmonary hypertension and multisystem organ failure.

○ **What is the advantage of pressure controlled ventilation in ARDS?**

It often allows for higher mean airway pressure with a lower peak airway pressure. Oxygenation often improves with an increase in the mean airway pressure.

○ **What are the three phases of ARDS?**

Acute or exudative, proliferative and fibrotic phase.

○ **What is the role of PEEP in ARDS?**

To maintain alveolar inflation and functional residual capacity. This optimizes V/Q matching and improves oxygenation.

○ **What are the negative effects of PEEP on cardiac output?**

PEEP may reduce cardiac output by reducing venous return, by increasing pulmonary vascular resistance and by shifting the interventricular septum to the left, thus reducing the left ventricular end diastolic volume.

○ **What are the ways that the optimal level of PEEP can be determined?**

Compliance, oxygenation, calculation of oxygen delivery and elucidation of the lower inflection point on the volume-pressure curve.

○ **What is the role of corticosteriods in ARDS?**

Steroids have not been shown effective in the early phase of ARDS. In the later stages of ARDS, steroids may have a role by reducing lung fibrosis.

○ **What interventions have been shown to reduce the mortality of ARDS?**

There never has been a clinically useful interventional study completed in adults that has clearly demonstrated an improved mortality in ARDS.

○ **Which drugs can cause ARDS?**

Opiates, salicylates, cocaine, protamine and certain chemotherapeutic agents.

○ **How long after an initial insult does ARDS usually occur?**

12 to 72 hours.

○ **What does ARDS stand for?**

Acute Respiratory Distress Syndrome is a better term than Adult Respiratory Distress Syndrome as this syndrome occurs in children.

○ **What is the characteristic histologic change in ARDS?**

Pathologists call this diffuse alveolar damage. It is characterized by a process of diffuse lung inflammation that progresses to fibrosis. Interestingly, the number of inflammatory cells observed is not large. There is heterogeneity both in time and space as to which alveoli are in the inflammatory phase and which are in the fibrotic phase. Another name for ARDS is hyaline membrane disease, which refers to the hyaline membranes seen histopathologically. These are collections of sloughed type 1 pneumocytes and other cellular debris.

○ **In patients diagnosed with ARDS, what are the most common causes of death?**

Multisystem organ failure or sepsis syndrome, not respiratory failure.

○ **T/F: Any cause of shock can cause ARDS.**

True.

○ **T/F: Too much oxygen can cause ARDS.**

True.

○ **What is a safe level of oxygen for prolonged use?**

An FiO_2 of 0.50 is safe and 0.60 is probably safe.

○ **T/F: A patient with ARDS can have a fever without having a source of infection.**

True.

○ **What is in the differential diagnosis of ARDS?**

Broadly three categories - cardiogenic pulmonary edema, pneumonia (PCP, fungi, bacteria, legionella, miliary TB) and inflammatory lung conditions (drug reaction, collagen vascular disease, BOOP, acute eosinophilic pneumonia).

○ **What is the optimal fluid management strategy in ARDS?**

No such strategy has been clearly demonstrated as the preferred strategy. Current thinking is to avoid hypervolemia while maintaining an adequate intravascular volume to optimize oxygen transport to peripheral organs.

○ **What is the current ventilator strategy in ARDS utilizing the lower and upper inflection points?**

To give enough PEEP to exceed the lower inflection point, thereby minimizing sheer forces on alveoli that results from the atelectatic alveoli being excessively opened and closed. This has an additional benefit of optimizing oxygenation by keeping the atelectatic alveoli open. The second component is to minimize the lung volume by keep the peak pressure below the upper inflection point, thereby avoiding overdistention of the alveoli.

This strategy makes pathophysiological sense but has not been clinically demonstrated to be clearly advantageous. Clinical trials are underway.

○ **What is permissive hypercapnia?**

The ventilator strategy of protecting the lungs from alveolar overdistention by reducing lung volumes and accepting, as a cost, the rise in pCO_2 and fall in pH. This is a controversial strategy, although two consensus conferences suggested that this strategy be utilized when plateau pressures are elevated. Studies are underway which will hopefully resolve the controversy.

O   **What is the plateau pressure? What is the peak airway pressure?**

The plateau pressure is the static pressure that exists when, at end inspiration, the airway is occluded. Occlusion of the airway creates a static column of air from the endotracheal tube to the alveoli. Because a static column of air is in pressure equilibrium, the pressure measured at the endotracheal tube is the same as that in the alveoli. The plateau pressure is a method to measure the alveolar distending pressure. An excessive elevation of this pressure is thought to reflect alveolar overdistention.

Peak airway pressure is the maximal excursion of the airway pressure gauge during the inspiratory and expiratory cycle.

O   **Does inverse ratio ventilation improve oxygenation in ARDS? Does it improve mortality?**

Inverse ratio ventilation is the strategy to reverse the normal 1:2 inspiration to expiration ratio in spontaneous breathing. This has been shown to improve oxygenation by increasing mean airway pressure at a lower peak pressure. The controversy is whether it has any beneficial effect over simply increasing PEEP. It is unknown if this strategy improves mortality.

O   **What is the effect of PEEP on right ventricular preload and afterload? How about on left ventricular preload and afterload?**

PEEP decreases preload to both ventricles, increases RV afterload and decreases LV afterload.

O   **Why does PEEP improve oxygen exchange in ARDS?**

PEEP reverses atelectasis and redistributes lung water from the alveoli to the interstitium.

O   **How does prone positioning improve oxygenation in ARDS?**

Prone positioning recruits dorsal lung units and improves V/Q matching.

O   **Are there any side effects noted with prone positioning?**

Yes. Although unusual, hypotension, desaturation and arrhythmias have occurred after prone positioning.

O   **What level is suggested as the maximal transalveolar pressure (as estimated by the plateau pressure) that will avoid barotrauma in a patient with ARDS?**

35 cm H_2O is commonly suggested in the literature. A recent editorial suggested that higher levels may be acceptable. Randomized trials addressing this are ongoing.

O   **What is the equation for the A-a gradient?**

A-a $= ((713 \text{ mmHg} \times FIO_2) - pCO_2/.8 - pO_2)$

The normal A-a gradient is 5 to 15 mmHg. The A-a gradient increases with pulmonary embolism.

O   **Most pulmonary emboli arise from what veins?**

The iliac and femoral veins.

○   **What is Virchow's triad?**

1) Injury to the endothelium of the vessels.
2) Hypercoagulable state.
3) Stasis.

○   **A 48 year old woman is transferred from another hospital a week and a half after sustaining a left upper extremity fracture, a complex pelvic fracture, bilateral lower extremity femur fractures and a left tibial fracture. While sitting in bed, she experiences severe dyspnea, tachypnea and tachycardia. Pulse oximetry reveals an oxygen saturation of 88% on room air. She is given supplemental oxygen and transferred to the ICU. What is your diagnosis?**

Pulmonary embolism secondary to deep vein thrombosis.

○   **What risk factors for deep vein thrombosis did she have?**

Trauma or surgery of pelvis or lower extremities, indwelling vascular catheters and prolonged immobility.

○   **What preventative measures can be taken in patients at risk for developing DVTs?**

Early ambulation, elastic stockings that provide graded compression from ankle to thigh, low-dose heparin, intermittent pneumatic compression and prophylactic inferior vena cava filters.

○   **What tests can be used to diagnosis pulmonary embolism?**

Pulmonary angiogram is the gold standard. V/Q (ventilation/perfusion) scans are the best non-invasive tests to establish or exclude the diagnosis of PE. A high probability scan in a clinical scenario of high likelihood for PE is an indication to treat. An intermediate or low probability scan necessitates further studies. Duplex ultrasound is used to detect DVT not to diagnose PE. However, if the duplex ultrasound is positive, then therapy for DVT will also treat PE.

○   **What are the indications for vena cava filter placement?**

Contraindication to anticoagulation, hemorrhage after anticoagulation, failure of anticoagulation to prevent recurrent pulmonary embolism and prophylaxis for extremely high-risk patients.

○   **What is the diagnostic test of choice for documenting DVT?**

Duplex ultrasound. The accuracy of physical examination for DVT is generally quoted to be 50%.

○   **What are the risk factors for DVT?**

Surgery (knee and hip greater than abdominal and urological)
Pregnancy
Cardiac disease, especially post-MI
Age greater than 50 years
Prior DVT
Immobilizaton
Acute paraplegia (but not chronic paraplegia)
Oral contraceptives (but not hormonal replacement therapy)
Major trauma

Malignancy, especially adenocarcinoma
Factor deficiency state
Antiphospholipid antibodies
Nephrotic syndrome
Paroxysmal nocturnal hemoglobinuria
Protein losing enteropathy

O   **Which factor deficiency states predispose to DVT?**

Activated protein C resistance
Protein C deficiency
Protein S deficiency
Plasminogen deficiency
Antithrombin III deficiency

O   **What are the symptoms of a PE?**

Dyspnea, pleurisy, cough, hemoptysis and syncope.

O   **What are the signs of PE?**

Crackles, increased P2, thrombophlebitis, heart gallop, peripheral edema, cardiac murmur and cyanosis.

O   **What is the goal for heparin therapy?**

To maintain the PTT between 1.5 and 2.5 times control.

O   **What is the goal for coumadin therapy?**

To maintain the INR between 2 and 3.

O   **What is the best initial method for localizing hemoptysis in a patient who is actively bleeding?**

Bronchoscopy.

O   **What is the location for aspiration pneumonias?**

In the supine patient, it is in the posterior segment of the upper lobe and in the superior segment of the lower lobe. In the upright patient, it is in the basilar segments of the lower lobes. The right lung is favored over the left because of the straighter takeoff of the right mainstem bronchus.

O   **What are the common directly toxic (non-infected) respiratory tract aspirates?**

Gastric contents, alcohol, hydrocarbons, mineral oil, animal and vegetable fats. All of these produce an inflammatory response and pneumonia. Gastric contents are the most common offender.

O   **What are the consequences of aspirating acid?**

The response is rapid, with near immediate bronchitis, bronchiolitis, atelectasis, shunting and hypoxemia. Pulmonary edema may occur within 4 hours. The clinical manifestations are dyspnea, wheezing, cough, cyanosis, fever and shock.

O   **What is the main priority in treating gastric acid aspiration?**

Maintenance of oxygenation. Intubation, ventilation and PEEP (positive end expiratory pressure) may be required.

○ **What are the radiographic manifestations of acid aspiration?**

Varied. There may be bilateral diffuse infiltrates, irregular "patchy" infiltrates or lobar infiltrates.

○ **What outcomes occur in patients who do not rapidly resolve gastric acid aspiration pneumonitis?**

ARDS (adult respiratory distress syndrome), progressive respiratory failure and bacterial superinfection.

○ **What is the predominant oropharyngeal flora in outpatients?**

Anaerobes. Community acquired aspiration is usually anaerobic. The most common aerobes involved are streptococcal species.

○ **What is the antibiotic of choice for outpatient acquired infectious aspiration pneumonia?**

Clindamycin.

○ **What is the bacteriology of inpatient acquired infectious aspiration pneumonia?**

Mixed aerobic and anaerobic organisms. Unlike outpatients, *Staphylococcus aureus*, *Escherichia coli*, *Pseudomonas aeruginosa* and *Proteus* species are common.

○ **What are the major causes of massive hemoptysis?**

Tuberculosis, bronchiectasis and lung cancer.

○ **What causes hemoptysis in patients with tuberculosis (either active or healed)?**

Pulmonary artery (Rasmussen's) aneurysm, bronchiolar ulceration and necrosis, bronchiectasis, broncholithiasis and mycetoma (fungus ball).

○ **What is the purpose of bronchoscopy in hemoptysis?**

Localization and diagnosis.

○ **What are the invasive therapies for massive hemoptysis?**

Thoracotomy, embolization, balloon tamponade (via bronchoscopy), double-lumen tube for lung separation and independent ventilation and laser bronchoscopy.

○ **When is surgery indicated for massive hemoptysis?**

Localized massive hemoptysis unresponsive to other therapy or electively, after stabilization, for long term control of localized bleeding.

○ **What are the major cardiovascular causes of hemoptysis?**

Mitral stenosis, pulmonary hypertension and Eisenmenger's complex.

○ **How does pulmonary artery catheterization produce hemoptysis?**

By pulmonary artery rupture, aneurysm formation and leakage and pulmonary infarction.

○ **What is a common definition for massive hemoptysis?**

Coughing of more than 600 ml of blood in 24 hours.

○ **What are the expected blood gas findings of a near-drowning victim?**

Metabolic acidosis from poor perfusion and hypoxia.

○ **Liquids pass from stomach to duodenum in 2 hours. Solids pass from stomach to duodenum in _____.**

4 to 6 hours

○ **What may delay gastric emptying?**

Anxiety, pain, drugs, diabetes mellitus, gastric outlet obstruction and pregnancy.

○ **Under what circumstances is aspiration of vomitus, oral secretions or foreign material likely?**

Anything resulting in an altered level of consciousness (e.g., alcohol, overdose, general anesthesia and stroke), impaired swallowing, abnormal gastrointestinal motility or disruption of esophageal sphincter function.

○ **T/F: Nasogastric tubes increase the risk of aspiration.**

True.

○ **What are the consequences of aspirating small (non-obstructing) food particles?**

Inflammation and hypoxemia that may result in chronic bronchiolitis or granulomatosis.

○ **What non-invasive bedside maneuver may assist management of massive hemoptysis?**

Positioning the bleeding lung in a dependent position

○ **How does hemoptysis differ from hematemesis?**

Blood in hemoptysis is often frothy and bright red. Alveolar macrophages may be seen on microscopy. Hematemesis is often acidic with a pH less than 2.5

○ **What is the major complication of a double lumen tube for independent lung ventilation?**

The tube may slip distally, such that no ventilation is provided to one lung or proximally, so that separation of the 2 sides is lost.

○ **Name some processes that cause the work of breathing to increase markedly in patients with COPD.**

Increased dead space ventilation requiring a higher minute ventilation, decreased respiratory muscle efficiency due to hyperinflation and increased airway resistance.

○   **Which pulmonary function tests increase in COPD?**

Residual volume and total lung capacity. All other tests (FEV_1, FEV_1/FVC, $FEV_{25-75\%}$ and DLCO) decrease.

○   **What is the risk of placing a patient with COPD on a high FIO_2?**

Suppression of the hypoxic ventilatory drive.

○   **What two diseases are usually seen in patients with COPD?**

Chronic bronchitis and emphysema.

○   **What are the risks of positive pressure mechanical ventilation?**

Ventilator-associated pneumonia, pulmonary barotrauma, hypotension and laryngotracheal complications.

○   **Has noninvasive positive pressure ventilation been shown to improve clinical outcome in acute exacerbation of COPD?**

Yes. Some studies have shown improved survival and hospital stay.

○   **Is a patient with an acute COPD exacerbation and impaired mental status a good candidate for a trial of noninvasive ventilation?**

No. Impaired mental status makes success less likely with noninvasive ventilation.

○   **Does noninvasive ventilation decrease the staffing requirements for treatment of respiratory failure in COPD?**

No. Experience and extensive training of physicians, nurses and respiratory care practitioners is required to maintain the necessary supervision of patients managed with noninvasive positive pressure ventilation.

○   **Can patients with COPD be successfully extubated without a weaning period?**

Yes. Many patients with COPD who undergo mechanical ventilation for acute bronchospasm, fluid overload, oversedation or inadvertent hyperoxygenation may be successfully extubated without weaning.

○   **What are the currently available techniques for weaning patients with COPD from mechanical ventilation?**

Assist-control ventilation with T-piece trials, synchronized intermittent mandatory ventilation and pressure support ventilation.

○   **What is the approximate FIO_2 delivered via nasal cannula at 2 liters per minute?**

$FIO_2 = 21\% + (2$ to 4 x oxygen liter flow$) = 25$ to 29%.

○   **What are the 3 major pathophysiological components of airway obstruction in asthma?**

Airway wall thickening from chronic inflammation and edema, mucus plugging and bronchoconstriction.

O   **What are the historical risk factors for status asthmaticus?**

Chronic steroid-dependent asthma
Prior ICU admission
Prior intubation
Recurrent ER visits in past 48 hours
Sudden onset of severe respiratory distress
Poor therapy compliance
Poor clinical recognition of attack severity
Hypoxic seizures

O   **What should be reserved for refractory status asthmaticus after the patient has been intubated?**

Halothane anesthesia produces prompt bronchodilation, but is difficult to administer and is reserved for the most severe cases.

O   **What are the criteria for ICU admission in a severe asthma case?**

PEFR < 30% baseline
PCO_2 > 40 mmHg
O_2 saturation < 90%
Severe obstruction with evidence of decreased air movement
Pulsus paradoxus >15 mmHg.

O   **What method of ventilation has been recently touted as a safe way to ventilate asthmatic patients with severe obstuction?**

Permissive hypercapnia. The acceptance of mild respiratory acidosis (to 7.20) to avoid high airway pressures is thought to reduce the incidence of hypotension and pneumothorax. With this strategy, lung volumes and the respiratory rate are reduced. A reduced respiratory rate permits more time for exhalation and prevents auto-PEEP. A reduction in lung volume also prevents auto-PEEP while reducing the peak airway pressure.

O   **What is the treatment for angioneurotic edema due to ACE inhibitors?**

Epinephrine, antihistamines and corticosteroids.

O   **What are the characteristics of bronchiolitis obliterans (obliterative bronchiolitis)?**

Stenosis of the bronchiolar lumen that results from chronic inflammation, scarring and smooth muscle hypertrophy.

O   **What are the most common causes of bronchiolitis obliterans?**

Toxic fume inhalation, viral, mycoplasma and legionella infection, bone marrow transplantation, lung transplantation (form of chronic rejection), rheumatoid arthritis, penicillamine, lupus, dermatomyositis and polymyositis.

O   **Does incentive spirometry prevent post-operative pulmonary function abnormalities?**

No. However, complications are reduced.

❍ What are the common pulmonary complications after upper abdominal surgery?

Atelectasis, bronchitis, cough, pneumonia, pleural effusion and respiratory failure.

❍ What studies best predict the risk of post-operative pulmonary complications?

Arterial blood gases and spirometry. CO_2 retention, FEV_1 less than 70% of predicted, FVC less than 70% of predicted and MVV less than 50% of predicted indicate high risk.

❍ How is lung function assessed prior to lung resection?

Spirometry and blood gas. If FEV_1 is greater than 2 liters or 80% predicted of normal and pCO_2 less than 45 mmHg, then no further testing is required.

❍ Why do we care about post-operative atelectasis?

If it persists for more than 72 hours, pneumonia may develop. Perioperative mortality rates are then 20%. Incentive spirometry is an important therapy for the prevention of atelectasis.

❍ What is the Vital Capacity (VC)?

It is the maximal volume of air expired from a maximal inspiratory level. It can be measured during a forced expiratory effort (FVC) or a more relaxed expiration (usually denoted as VC or SVC). The VC and FVC should be equal in a normal, non-obstructed patient. In patients with obstructive diseases the FVC is generally lower than the VC/SVC.

❍ What is the FEV_1?

The FEV_1 is perhaps the single most important spirometric value. It is the volume of air expired in the first second of an FVC maneuver. It can be expressed as an absolute value or as a percentage of the FVC (FEV_1/FVC ratio).

❍ What is a normal FEV_1?

It is usually interpreted in the context of established predicted normal mean values. A normal FEV_1 is a value greater than 80% of predicted normal.

❍ What is maximal voluntary ventilation (MVV)?

This is a maneuver where the patient is asked to breathe as rapidly and deeply as possible over a 12 second period. Exhaled volume is measured and extrapolated over a minute and is expressed in liters per minute. This test provides an overall assessment of pulmonary function, including respiratory muscle strength.

❍ What is the relationship between FEV_1 and MVV?

The MVV is usually 35 to 40 times the FEV_1.

❍ What is "small airways disease"?

This term refers to obstructive disease localized to peripheral airways with diameters 2 mm or smaller. Small airway disease is characterized by decrement in FEF $_{25-75\%}$, which correlates with airflow in the middle 50% of VC maneuver and is effort independent.

O   **What are the most common causes of restrictive pulmonary physiology?**

Parenchymal lung disease (e.g. pulmonary fibrosis), pleural disease (e.g. fibrothorax), neuromuscular disease and thoracic cage abnormalities (e.g. kyphoscoliosis).

O   **What is the functional residual capacity (FRC)?**

The volume of air remaining in the lungs after a normal expiration. It is measured with the patient's glottis open to atmosphere.

O   **What is total lung lapacity (TLC)?**

The volume of air in the lungs after a maximal inspiration. It represents the sum of all volume compartments in the lungs.

O   **What is a normal TLC?**

Values between 80 and 120% of established predicted normal mean values.

O   **What is the residual volume (RV)?**

The volume of air remaining in the lungs after a maximal expiration. It represents the difference between FRC and expiratory reserve volume (ERV) or the maximal volume of air expired from a resting end-expiratory level.

O   **What is a normal RV?**

Values between 80 and 120% of established predicted normal mean values.

O   **The diagnosis of a restrictive pattern requires a decrement in which lung volume?**

Total lung capacity (TLC). While a reduction in FEV_1 and FVC, with a normal FEV_1/FVC ratio may suggest restriction, the diagnosis of restriction is based on a decreased TLC. The assessment of the severity of restriction is also based on the TLC.

O   **Which pulmonary function value best predicts prognosis/mortality in COPD?**

The FEV_1.

O   **What are maximal inspiratory and expiratory pressures (MIP, MEP)?**

Specific tests of respiratory muscle function. Pressures generated by maximal inspiratory and expiratory efforts are measured by a pressure gauge.

O   **What is the definition of normal pulmonary function?**

Normal pH, PCO_2 and PO_2, without excessive pulmonary or cardiac work.

O   **How are the lung volumes altered in patients with severe obstructive disease?**

The RV and TLC are increased, indicating hyperinflation.

○ **What is a normal tidal volume?**

500 cc.

○ **What is a normal amount of anatomic dead space?**

150 cc.

○ **What is a normal minute ventilation?**

7,500 cc/min.

○ **What is the intrapleural pressure in the case of a pneumothorax?**

It is zero in a non-tension pneumothorax at end expiration. The lung collapses because of the intrinsic elastic properties of the lung. The intrapleural pressure is positive in the case of a tension pneumothorax.

○ **Differentiate between transudate and exudate.**

Transudate: effusion to serum protein ratio is < 0.5 and for LDH the ratio is < 0.60. Also, the effusion LDH is < 2/3 of the upper limit of normal for LDH. Most commonly occurs with CHF, renal disease and liver disease.

Exudate: effusion to serum protein ratio is > 0.5 and for LDH the ratio is > 0.6. The effusion LDH is > 2/3 of the upper limit of normal for LDH. Most commonly occurs with infections, malignancy and trauma.

○ **Why is supplemental oxygen recommended in the conservative treatment of pneumothorax?**

Absorption of a loculated pneumothorax is hastened by oxygen inhalation, which increases the pressure gradient of gases between the pleura and the capillaries.

○ **What is the most common cause of a large pleural effusion?**

Malignancy.

○ **What is the most common cause of a malignant pleural effusion?**

Carcinoma of the lung.

○ **What is the most common etiology of a spontaneous pneumothorax?**

Rupture of a pulmonary bleb.

○ **Which diseases are associated with pneumothorax?**

COPD, asthma, IPF, eosinophilic granuloma and lymphangioleiomyomatosis.

○ **Which types of pneumonia are commonly associated with pneumothorax?**

Staphylococcus, TB, klebsiella and PCP

O   **What is the indication for a tube thoracostomy in patients with a pneumothorax?**

Over 20 % pneumothorax or a clinical indication such as respiratory distress or enlarging pneumothorax.

O   **What special chest x-ray may be useful for diagnosing pneumothorax?**

An expiratory film.

O   **What is a chylothorax?**

It is a fluid collection in the pleural space due to disruption of the thoracic duct. Common causes include trauma related to cardiovascular surgery, lymphoma, Kaposi's sarcoma and other tumors. The fluid is milky and remains cloudy after centrifugation. The presence of chylomicrons verifies the diagnosis. If the fluid triglyceride level exceeds 110, then it is highly likely that a chylothorax is present. Treatment consists of spontaneous repair, pleuroperitoneal shunt, pleurodesis and duct ligation.

O   **What is a pseudochylothorax?**

It is a long standing pleural fluid collection in which the fluid has become chyliform. The presence of cholesterol crystals verifies the diagnosis. A fluid cholesterol level above 250 suggests the diagnosis. The most common causes of this effusion are TB and RA.

O   **What is a hemothorax?**

It is when the pleural fluid hematocrit is at least 50 % of that in the blood. All traumatic hemothoraces should have chest tube drainage. Thoracotomy is necessary for ongoing bleeding. Nontraumatic hemothorax is usually due to metastatic disease or as a complication to anticoagulation.

O   **What are the indications for the chest tube placement in parapneumonic effusion?**

Presence of a complicated parapneumonic effusion indicates the need for a chest tube. This is demonstrable by the gross appearance of purulent fluid (pus), bacterial on gram stain, positive culture of pleural fluid, low glucose (usually < 40 mg/dl), low pH (less than 7.0) and elevated LDH (>1000 IU/L; the LDH criterion alone is controversial).

O   **What are the characteristics of an effusion associated with pulmonary embolism?**

These may be transudative, exudative or hemorrhagic. The predominate cell type may be polymorphonuclear or mononuclear.

O   **What drugs are known to have caused bronchiolitis obliterans organizing pneumonia?**

Bleomycin, penicillamine, amiodarone, cocaine, cyclophosphamide, mitomycin C, methotrexate, sulfasalazine and gold.

O   **How is diaphragmatic paralysis treated?**

Usually unilateral involvement requires no treatment. Bilateral paralysis can be treated with mechanical ventilatory support (e.g., BiPAP, rocking bed or negative pressure ventilation).

O   **In low cervical and upper thoracic spinal injuries, the diaphragm is intact. What occurs to the cough mechanism?**

It is decreased because the expiratory muscles are innervated below C8.

○ **What diffuse neuromuscular diseases can cause respiratory muscle weakness and are acute in onset?**

Myasthenia gravis, Eaton-Lambert syndrome, organophosphate poisoning, botulism and aminoglycosides toxicity.

○ **What diffuse neuromuscular diseases can cause respiratory muscle weakness and are gradual in onset?**

ALS, muscular dystrophies and myopathies (e.g., alcohol and diabetes).

○ **What measurements should be assessed in these patients?**

Vital capacity and inspiratory and expiratory maximal pressures.

○ **Bronchiolitis obliterans may occur as a complication in which type of transplants?**

Bone marrow, heart-lung and lung transplantation.

○ **What are the most common causes of interstitial lung disease?**

In order: interstitial pulmonary fibrosis, collagen-vascular disease related, hypersensitivity pneumonitis, sarcoidosis, BOOP, eosinophilic granuloma and asbestosis.

○ **How is primary pulmonary hypertension (PPH) diagnosed?**

It is diagnosed after ruling out cardiac, pulmonary and other causes of pulmonary hypertension. A right heart catherization confirms the presence of pulmonary hypertension. Echocardiography is useful to noninvasivelly follow the disease progression. A V/Q scan is useful to rule out pulmonary embolism as a cause for the elevated pulmonary arterial pressures.

○ **What is the treatment for PPH?**

Oxygen, calcium channel blockers, prostacyclin (which can only be given intravenously) and anticoagulation. Inhaled nitric oxide is being studied.

○ **What are the causes of secondary pulmonary hypertension?**

Cardiac disease, interstitial lung disease, COPD, hypoventilation syndromes, collagen-vascular diseases, pulmonary emboli that went undetected, HIV infection and drugs as fenfluramine and aminorex.

○ **What is pulmonary veno-occlusive disease?**

It is characterized by pulmonary hypertension resulting from inflammation and thrombosis of the pulmonary veins and venules. The wedge pressure is often normal. The CXR may show signs of pulmonary edema without the pulmonary artery pruning seen in PPH. The diagnosis is made by catheterization and lung biopsy.

○ **What is the major etiology of pulmonary hypertension?**

Chronic hypoxia.

○   **What are the clinical features of fat embolism syndrome?**

It is characterized by hypoxemia, diffuse infiltrates, neurological abnormalities (confusion, seizures, coma, focal defects) and petechiae that appear on the head, neck and axillae. The syndrome usually occurs 24 to 72 hours after the inciting event.

○   **How is the fat embolism syndrome diagnosed?**

Clinically. There are no specific tests available. The presence of fat globules in the serum is neither sensitive nor specific.

○   **How is fat embolism syndrome treated?**

Supportively. There is no specific treatment. Some have suggested that corticosteroids are effective in preventing the occurance of the syndrome.

○   **Define apnea, hypopnea and apnea/hypopnea index.**

Apnea: cessation of airflow for at least 10 sec.
Hypopnea: decrement of 50% or more in airflow with consequent 4% or more fall in O_2 saturation or electroencephalographic arousal.
Apnea/hypopnea index: number of apneas and hypopneas per hour.

○   **What is the most likely cause of severe head, neck and arm swelling in a patient with a centrally located mass on chest radiograph?**

Superior vena cava syndrome, the partial or complete mechanical obstruction of the superior vena cava by an intrathoracic tumor or nodal metastases.

○   **Hypercalcemia in the absence of bony metastases is associated with which lung cancer?**

Squamous cell carcinoma (a paraneoplastic syndrome associated with tumor elaboration of a PTH-like substance).

○   **The syndrome of inappropriate secretion of antidiuretic hormone is associated with which cell type of lung cancer?**

Small cell carcinoma

○   **What does normal ventilation with decreased perfusion suggest?**

Pulmonary embolus (PE).

○   **What procedures should be performed to confine aspiration in a patient who is continuously vomiting and at risk for aspiration pneumonia?**

Lie the patient on his right side in the Trendelenburg position. This will help confine the aspiration to the right upper lobe.

○   **What is the most common postoperative respiratory complication?**

Atelectasis. Respiratory failure and aspiration pneumonia are other postoperative complications.

O   **In the elderly, what is the most common cause of death due to infection in the community, in institutions, and in the hospital?**

In the community and institutions, it is bacterial pneumonia; and in hospitals, it is UTIs.

O   **How do steroids function in the treatment of asthma?**

Steroids increase cAMP, decrease inflammation, and aid in restoring the function of □-adrenergic responsiveness to adrenergic drugs.

O   **Signs of tension pneumothorax on a physical exam include what?**

Tachypnea, unilateral absent breath sounds, tachycardia, pallor, diaphoresis, cyanosis, tracheal deviation, hypotension, and neck vein distention.

O   **What are the most common symptoms of a PE?**

Chest Pain (88%) and dyspnea (84%).

O   **When assisting an MD with a chest tube removal, how should you instruct the patient to breathe?**

Exhale deeply when the MD removes the tube.

O   **One hour after extubation, the physician orders arterial blood gasses and wants to be called if they are abnormal. The ABGs are as follows: pO$_2$: 90, pCO$_2$: 40, pH: 7.36. Should you notify the physician?**

No. These are normal.

O   **A client is admitted with pneumonia and the MD orders sputum cultures to be obtained before antibiotics are begun. The patient is unable to cough up any sputum. What should you do?**

Obtain an order to have a sputum sample induced with an aerosol treatment. If still unsuccessful, notify the MD.

O   **You note a cessation of fluctuation in the water seal bottle from a chest tube. What is the most likely cause?**

Chest tube obstruction.

O   **What is the mode of transmission for the tubercle bacillus?**

Inhalation of tubercle-laden droplets.

O   **Interpret the following blood gases: pH: 7.49, PaCO$_2$: 26, HCO$_3$: 23, PaO$_2$: 100.**

Respiratory alkalosis.

O   **Interpret the following blood gases: pH: 7.49, PaCO$_2$: 36, HCO$_3$: 40, PaO$_2$: 92.**

Metabolic alkalosis.

○   **Interpret the following blood gases: pH: 7:30, PaCO₂: 50, HCO₃: 24, PaO₂: 80.**

Respiratory Acidosis.

○   **Interpret the following blood gases: pH: 7:30, PaCO₂: 40, HCO₃: 20, PaO₂: 95.**

Metabolic Acidosis.

○   **You note that there is no bubbling in the suction compartment of the water seal container of a chest tube. What would be your best course of action?**

Check the order to see if the chest tube is ordered with suction and how much. If suction is ordered, increase the suction to the amount ordered.

○   **Why is the administration of propanolol hydrochloride (Inderal) used cautiously in clients with COPD?**

It can cause airway resistance.

○   **What type of lab study is used to determine if the tubercle bacilli is present in sputum?**

Acid-fast staining.

○   **Following a pulmonary lobectomy, you note a decrease in blood pressure, the patient is restless, short of breath, and the chest tube drainage has become sanguineous. What should you suspect?**

Possible internal bleeding at the surgical site.

○   **A client is admitted with pneumonia. Prior to starting antibiotics, what lab tests should you check?**

Check the results of all cultures obtained.

○   **One hour following extubation, a client's PaO₂ is 90 mm Hg. You would interpret this level as:**

Adequate. A normal range is 80-100 mm Hg.

○   **Following a lung lobectomy, you assess the incision line and feel a crackling sensation. What is this called?**

Subcutaneous emphysema.

○   **What should you do if you find subcutaneous emphysema?**

Keep track of its progression. If it spreads rapidly or involves the neck area, it should be reported. Otherwise it poses no danger and is normal after this type of surgery.

○   **What is a hallmark lab sign of ARDS (adult respiratory distress syndrome)?**

Refractory hypoxemia. The PaO₂ level continues to fall despite administering higher levels of oxygen.

○   **Following removal of a chest tube, what should be placed over the wound?**

A petrolatum gauze dressing.

○   **What type of breath sounds will you hear when a pneumothorax is present?**

No breath sounds.

○   **What is the purpose of aminophylline in a patient with COPD?**

To relax and dilate the bronchi and relive bronchial constriction and spasm.

○   **What level should the collection and suction bottles from a chest tube be kept at in relation to the patient?**

Below the level of the patient's chest.

○   **Above what level of oxygen concentration is there an increased risk for causing oxygen toxicity?**

40%.

○   **What conclusion can be drawn from a PaO_2 level of 50 in a client that exhibits no signs or symptoms of hypoxia?**

The arterial blood gas is not truly arterial.

○   **If a patient's pCO_2 level is high, what conclusion can you make about the patient?**

The patient is hypoventilating. This is generally the only cause of a high pCO_2.

○   **What is an early behavioral sign of hypoxia?**

Anxiety.

○   **What nerve has the potential to be damaged when a tracheostomy tube is in place?**

The laryngeal nerve.

○   **What is the most important nursing goal for a client with a new tracheostomy tube?**

Maintain a patent airway.

○   **What do crackles (rales) in the lungs indicate?**

The alveoli are filled with fluid.

○   **What is the most effective way to evaluate the effectiveness of tracheobronchial suctioning?**

Auscultate the lungs before and after the procedure.

○   **Following a laryngectomy, what is the priority nursing goal in the immediate post-op period?**

Maintain a patent airway.

❍   **Why would you hyper oxygenate a patient prior to suctioning his airway?**

To prevent hypoxia resulting from the suctioning procedure.

❍   **What solution may be instilled into a tracheostomy or endotracheal tube to help liquefy secretions prior to suctioning?**

1-2 ml of sterile normal saline.

❍   **What are the signs and symptoms of a pneumothorax?**

Tachypnea, restlessness, hypotension dyspnea, and possible hypoxia.

❍   **What is the most reliable and accurate way to administer oxygen to a patient with COPD?**

Venturi mask.

❍   **During the postoperative period, how often should a patient cough and deep breath?**

Every two hours.

❍   **When using one hand to ventilate an adult patient with an Ambu bag, how many cc's of air are delivered?**

400 cc.

❍   **When using two hands to ventilate with an Ambu bag, how much air can be delivered?**

1,000 cc of air.

❍   **What are some of the causes of a respiratory alkalosis?**

Pulmonary embolism, asthma, severe hypoxia, high fever, and hyperventilation syndrome.

❍   **What activities should you encourage a patient to do after he has had chest surgery?**

Sit upright and perform deep breathing and coughing exercises.

❍   **What is the most common site for a pulmonary emboli to originate?**

The leg veins.

❍   **What is Cheyne-Stokes respiration?**

Alternating periods of apnea and deep, rapid breathing.

❍   **What is the most common symptom of a pulmonary embolis?**

Chest pain.

GASTROINTESTINAL PEARLS

○ **What are the pulmonary manifestations of pancreatitis?**

Hypoxemia with normal CXR, ARDS and pleural effusions.

○ **Contrast acute versus chronic effusions associated with pancreatitis.**

Acute: occurs when abdominal symptoms are dominant and the effusion is small to moderate.
Chronic: occurs when abdominal symptoms have resolved, chest symptoms predominate and the effusion is large. It may be due to a fistula from the pancreas to the pleural space.

○ **What are the pulmonary manifestations of cirrhosis?**

Hypoxemia (due to V/Q mismatching and microvascular shunting), pleural effusions (transudative, usually right sided, usually associated with ascites), reduction in static lung volumes due to ascites and pulmonary hypertension.

○ **Prophylaxis for stress ulcers includes what agents?**

Sucralfate, antacids and histamine receptor antagonists.

○ **If blood is recovered from the stomach after an NG tube is inserted, where is the most likely location of the bleed?**

Above the ligament of Treitz.

○ **How much blood must be lost in the GI tract to cause melena?**

50 ml. Healthy patients normally lose 2.5 ml/day.

○ **What are the most common causes of upper GI bleeding?**

Ulcer disease (45%), esophageal varices (20%), gastritis (20%) and Mallory-Weiss syndrome (10%)

○ **What percentage of patients with upper GI bleeds will stop bleeding within hours of hospitalization?**

85%. About 25% of these patients will rebleed within the first 2 days of hospitalization. If no rebleeding occurs in five days, the chance of rebleeding is only 2%.

○ **What is the most common cause of portal hypertension?**

Intrahepatic obstruction (90%), which is most often due to cirrhosis.

○ **What is Charcot's triad?**

1) Fever

2) Jaundice
3) Abdominal pain
This is the hallmark of acute cholangitis.

O   **What is Reynolds' pentad?**

Charcot's triad plus shock and mental status changes. This is the hallmark of acute toxic ascending cholangitis.

O   **What are Ranson's criteria?**

A means of estimating prognosis for patients with pancreatitis.

At initial presentation	Developing within 24 hours
Age > 55 WBC > 16,000/mm^3 AST > 250 IU/L Serum glucose > 200 mg/dl LDH > 350	Hematocrit falling > 10% Increase in BUN > 5 mg/dl Serum Ca$^+$ < 8 mg/dl Arterial PO$_2$ < 60 mm Hg Base deficit > 4 mEq/L Fluid sequestration > 6000 ml

O   **Until discounted, what intra-abdominal pathology should be assumed for a pregnant woman with right upper quadrant pain?**

Acute appendicitis.

O   **Which method is more sensitive for locating the source of GI bleeding, a radioactive Tc-labeled red cell scan or angiography?**

A bleeding scan can detect a site bleeding at a rate as low as 0.1 ml/min., while angiography requires more rapid bleeding, at least 0.5 ml/min.

O   **Repeated violent bouts of vomiting can result in both Mallory-Weiss tears and Boerhaave's syndrome. What is the difference between the two?**

Mallory-Weiss tears: Involve the submucosa and mucosa, typically in the right posterolateral wall of the gastroesophageal junction.
Boerhaave's syndrome: A full-thickness tear, usually in the unsupported left posterolateral wall of the abdominal esophagus.

O   **What is the most frequent complication of choledocholithiasis?**

Cholangitis (60%). Other complications are bile duct obstruction, pancreatitis, biliary enteric fistula and hemobilia.

O   **A 22 year-old female with sickle-cell disease presents with fever, shaking chills and jaundice. What is the diagnosis?**

Charcot's triad suggests ascending cholangitis. The precipitating cause is probably pigment stones resulting from chronic hemolysis.

O   **A patient presents with palmar erythema, spider angiomas, testicular atrophy and asterixis. What other signs and symptoms may be exhibited?**

Hematemesis, encephalopathy, hepatomegaly, splenomegaly, jaundice, caput medusa, ascites and gynecomastia may also occur. This patient has cirrhosis.

O   **A cirrhotic patient vomits bright red blood and has a systolic blood pressure of 90 mm Hg. After aggressive fluid resuscitation with 4 units of packed RBCs and a gastric lavage, his pressure is still 90 mm Hg. What's next?**

Assume a coagulopathy. Transfuse fresh frozen plasma, start a vasopressin or octreotide drip and arrange for an emergent endoscopic evaluation/intervention, usually for sclerotherapy or banding.

O   **A cirrhotic patient presents with weakness and edema. What electrolyte imbalances might be present?**

Hyponatremia (dilutional or diuretic induced), hypokalemia (from GI losses or diuretics) and hypomagnesemia.

O   **What diuretic is the optimal choice for cirrhotic patients with ascites?**

Potassium sparing agents. These medications treat the hyperaldosterone state specifically.

O   **A 73 year-old woman with no prior medical history presents with fever, chills, vomiting, nausea and an acute onset of pain in her left lower quadrant. Her pain becomes worse after she eats and is mildly relieved after a bowel movement. Upon physical examination, you note that she has guarding, rebound tenderness and a tender, firm, non-mobile mass in the left lower quadrant. What is the most likely diagnosis?**

Diverticulitis.

O   **Which type of hepatitis is characterized by an SPGT greater than the SGOT?**

Viral hepatitis. The SGPT is usually greater than 1,000.

O   **Which type of hepatitis is usually contracted through blood transfusions?**

Hepatitis C accounts for 85% of hepatitis infections via this route.

O   **List four contraindications to the introduction of a nasogastric tube.**

1) Suspected esophageal laceration or perforation
2) Near obstruction due to stricture
3) Esophageal foreign body
4) Severe head trauma with rhinorrhea

O   **What test should be performed when an elderly patient is suffering from pain that is out of proportion to the physical examination?**

Angiography. This test is the gold standard for diagnosing mesenteric ischemia.

O   **What is the most frequent cause of small bowel obstruction?**

Adhesions, followed by incarcerated hernias, are the most common causes of extraluminal obstruction. Gallstones and bezoars are the most common causes of intraluminal obstruction.

O   **Is a serum amylase test or a lipase test more specific for pancreatitis?**

Lipase.

O   **Is a nasogastric tube always required for acute pancreatitis?**

No, only if nausea and vomiting are severe. In fact, one study showed that NG tubes contributed to more complications, including aspiration.

O   **What is the most common cause of lower GI perforation?**

Diverticulitis, followed by tumor, colitis, foreign bodies and instrumentation.

O   **What are some indications for surgery in a bleeding ulcer?**

A visible vessel in the ulcer bed, more than 6 units of blood transfused in 24 hours or more than 3 to 4 units transfused per day for three days.

O   **Are "stress ulcers" a surgical problem?**

Typically not. The diffuse gastric bleeding that results from CNS tumors, head trauma, burns, sepsis, shock, steroids, aspirin or alcohol is usually mucosal and can be life threatening. However, this condition can usually be managed medically. Endoscopic diagnosis is key.

O   **What medical conditions are related to an increased incidence of peptic ulcers?**

COPD, cirrhosis and chronic renal failure.

O   **What is the treatment for pseudomembranous colitis?**

Oral metronidazole (preferred) or vancomycin.

O   **What is a pancreatic pseudocyst?**

Collection of necrotic tissue, fluid and blood that develops without a true capsule. It develops over a period of 1 to 4 weeks.

O   **What are the most common causes of colonic obstruction?**

Cancer, then diverticulitis followed by volvulus.

O   **In a patient with pancreatitis, what complications are suggested by symptoms that last longer than a week or an abdominal mass with leukocytosis?**

Pancreatic abscess or pseudocyst.

O   **What is abdominal compartment syndrome?**

Increased pressure within the confined anatomical space of the abdomen that may impair end organ perfusion and physiologic function.

O   **What is the most common cause of intra-abdominal compartment syndrome?**

Coagulopathy with post-operative intra-abdominal hemorrhage.

O   **What is the treatment for leaking ascites following major surgery?**

Return to the operating room for repair of fascial dehiscence.

O   **What is the difference between fascial dehiscence and evisceration?**

Facial dehiscence involves separation of the closed fascia with or without evisceration of the bowel. Evisceration is a surgical emergency.

O   **What is the most common cause of fascial dehiscence?**

Intra-abdominal sepsis.

O   **Forty eight hours post-operatively, a patient develops severe pain about his midline wound, skin bullae, crepitus and irregular blanching at the wound margins with a fever of 104. What is the most likely diagnosis?**

Clostridial gas gangrene.

O   **What is the most appropriate initial therapy for a patient with bleeding esophageal varices?**

Octreotide (somatostatin analogue) infusion. Vasopressin along with nitroglycerin (to offset the coronary vasoconstriction caused by vasopressin) can be used if this is unavailable. Any coagulation defect must be corrected.

O   **What are the other non-surgical options for bleeding esophageal varices that do not respond to somatostatin infusion?**

Placement of Sengstaken-Blakemore tube, sclerotherapy or banding of varices and transjugular intrahepatic portosystemic shunting.

O   **Four days following placement of a percutaneous endoscopic gastrostomy tube a patient develops sudden onset of fever, chills, tachycardia and hypotension. Physical exam shows abdominal distention and plain films show a large amount of free air. The most likely cause is?**

Gastric leakage due to necrosis.

O   **What is the most feared complication following duodenal surgery?**

Duodenal fistula with intra-abdominal sepsis.

O   **What is the risk of tube feeding a patient with an ileus?**

Massive small bowel necrosis. This unusual complication is seen primarily in critically ill patients and has an unclear etiology.

O   **What procedure should a patient with a bowel obstruction and sigmoid volvulus undergo?**

Attempted colonoscopic decompression, either with a rigid or flexible endoscope. If this is unsuccessful the patient will require laparotomy with sigmoid colectomy.

O   **What intravenous antibiotic is effective in treating Clostridium difficile associated with an ileus?**

Metronidazole.

O   **What is the appropriate surgical therapy for toxic Clostridium difficile colitis?**

Total colectomy with end ileostomy.

O   **What disease is suggested by Grey-Turner's sign (flank ecchymosis) and Cullen's sign (periumbilical ecchymosis)?**

Severe necrotizing pancreatitis with retroperitoneal hemorrhage.

O   **Five days following splenectomy for trauma a patient is diagnosed with a subphrenic abscess. Fluid from a percutaneous drainage reveals the amylase to be 48,000.   What is the diagnosis?**

Pancreatic fistula.   The tail of the pancreas was likely injured during the splenectomy.

O   **A patient admitted to the ICU for shock describes terrible abdominal pain out of proportion to their physical exam. What is the most likely diagnosis?**

Intestinal infarction.

O   **Following infrarenal aortic replacement for aneurysmal disease, a patient becomes hypotensive with worsening abdominal distention. What is the next appropriate step?**

Immediate return to the operating room for repair of vascular suture line dehiscence.

O   **A patient with a type B thoracic aortic aneurysm admitted to the ICU for medical treatment develops oliguria, increased fluid requirements and acute abdominal pain 24 hours later. What is the most likely explanation?**

Extension of the dissection with compromise of intestinal perfusion.

O   **What is the mechanism of necrosis and vascular damage in acute pancreatitis?**

Autodigestion of the pancreas by various proteolytic and lipolytic enzymes.

O   **Is mesenteric ischemia more serious in the small or large bowel?**

The small bowel. Embolization in the superior mesenteric artery effects the entire small bowel. Embolization to the large bowel is not as serious due to collateral circulation to the large bowel.

O   **Which common electrolyte disturbances occur in patients who have acute pancreatitis?**

Hypocalcemia and hypomagnesemia.

O   **What are Grey-Turner's and Cullen's signs?**

Grey-Turner's sign: Flank ecchymosis indicative of pancreatic disease.
Cullen's sign : Periumbilical ecchymosis indicative of pancreatic disease.
Both are caused by dissection of blood retroperitoneally.

○ **List four contraindications to the introduction of a nasogastric tube.**

Suspected esophageal laceration or perforation, near obstruction due to stricture, esophageal foreign body, and severe head trauma with rhinorrhea.

○ **APAP (acetaminophen) poisoning can produce damage to which internal organ?**

The liver.

○ **What is the most common cause of abdominal pain in the elderly?**

Constipation.

○ **What is the most common cause of paralytic ileus?**

Surgery.

○ **What is the incubation period for hepatitis A?**

30 days. An RNA virus causes this disease.

○ **How is hepatitis A transmitted?**

By the oral fecal route. No carrier state exists.

○ **What symptoms would you expect to find in a patient who has a perforated duodenal ulcer?**

Abdominal rigidity and tenderness.

○ **Following a subtotal gastrectomy, what is the purpose of setting the NG tube to low intermittent suction?**

To prevent pressure on the suture lines from accumulated gas or fluid.

○ **What is the preferred way to determine if a nasogastric tube has been correctly inserted?**

Apply suction to the tube and observe for the return of stomach contents, and instill air into the tube while auscultating over the epigastric area.

○ **What stool color indicates that a patient has bleeding in his upper GI tract?**

Black.

○ **Why would a patient with a common bile duct obstruction be monitored for prolonged bleeding?**

Because if bleeding is present, bile is prevented from entering the intestinal tract, thus preventing the absorption of fat soluble vitamins such as vitamin K, which is necessary for prothrombin formation.

❍   **In a subtotal gastrectomy (Billroth II), the stomach contents will bypass what anatomical structure?**

The duodenum and go directly to the jejunum.

❍   **Following a subtotal gastrectomy, what type of drainage would you expect from the NGT immediately post-op?**

Some bright red bloody drainage, but not in large amounts.

❍   **What lab value would be elevated in a patient with pancreatitis?**

Serum amylase and lipase.

❍   **What nursing measure can help alleviate a sore nares when a nasogastric tube is in place?**

Applying a water-soluble lubricant around the tube.

❍   **How long should you listen in each quadrant to confirm the absence of bowel sounds?**

5 minutes.

❍   **What type of solution should be used to irrigate a nasogastric tube and why?**

Normal saline. Usage of hypotonic or hypertonic solutions could cause electrolyte imbalances.

❍   **What is the purpose of a Sengstaken-Blakemore tube?**

Used in treating esophageal varices, this tube has a gastric balloon that anchors and applies pressure to the cardiac sphincter and a larger esophageal balloon that that applies pressure to the bleeding sites in the esophagus. Aspiration of stomach contents with a syringe and irrigation is still possible.

❍   **What is the physiological reason for the development of ascites in cirrhosis?**

Portal hypertension and low levels of serum albumin leading to decreased colloidal osmotic pressure and sodium retention, thus fluid leaves the intravascular space and collects in the interstitial space.

❍   **What is the danger of the gastric balloon rupturing or deflating in a Sengstaken-Blakemore tube?**

The esophageal balloon can move up, obstructing the airway.

❍   **What is the purpose of lactulose (Chronulac) administration in cirrhosis?**

It decreases ammonia formation in the intestine by increasing intestinal motility and causing diarrhea.

❍   **A patient with ascites would receive serum albumin for what purpose?**

To increase the colloidal osmotic pressure so fluid will flow from the tissues back into the intravascular space.

❍   **What effect would you see if the administration of serum albumin has been successful?**

An increase in urine output as fluid leaves the tissues and returns to the plasma.

○   **What is purpose of administering oral neomycin and/or neomycin enemas to a patient who has cirrhosis?**

The neomycin helps decrease the amount of bacteria in the intestines. This will produce ammonia as a by-product of digested blood.

○   **What is portal systemic encephalopathy?**

A toxic effect on the central nervous system resulting from the liver's inability to detoxify ammonia.

○   **What are Curling's ulcers?**

Stress ulcers that can develop as a result of physiological stress from a burn. The chance of these ulcers developing is usually proportional to the extent of the burn.

○   **What are the signs and symptoms of a perforated peptic ulcer?**

Sudden severe upper abdominal pain, vomiting and a tender rigid abdomen.

○   **What are the signs and symptoms of a small bowel obstruction?**

Decreased bowel sounds, abdominal distention, decreased flatus, and projectile vomiting.

○   **What is the most common postoperative problem?**

Bleeding.

GENITOURINARY/RENAL PEARLS

○ **What is the most common infectious cause of the hemolytic uremic syndrome?**

E. coli (O157:H7).

○ **What is the prognosis for patients with acute renal failure secondary to HUS?**

Over 90% survival with many patients eventually recovering normal renal function.

○ **What are the pulmonary manifestations of chronic renal disease?**

Pulmonary edema, pleural effusions, uremic pleuritis, metastatic calcifications, urinothorax, pO_2 reduction during hemodialysis and atelectasis associated with peritoneal dialysis.

○ **What is the mechanism for pO_2 reduction during hemodialysis?**

The primary mechanism is hypoventilation due to decreased CO_2 production that is associated with the oxidation of acetate. Secondarily, complement is activated resulting in leukocyte and platelet aggregation, which alters V/Q.

○ **A patient with polyuria, low urine osmolality and high serum osmolality is given vasopressin. No change in osmolality is noted. Which type of diabetes insipidus (DI) does she have?**

Nephrogenic. The distal renal tubules are refractory to antidiuretic hormone.

○ **What are the indications for emergency hemodialysis?**

Elevated potassium with ECG changes, decreased pH, pericarditis, mental status changes and severe volume overload.

○ **What is the etiology of acute renal failure seen a few weeks after cardiac catheterization?**

Cholesterol emboli syndrome.

○ **What treatments are used to ameliorate bleeding in a uremic patient?**

Dialysis, DDAVP, cryoprecipitate or platelet transfusions.

○ **What are the most common cause of acute renal failure seen after repair of an abdominal aneurysm?**

Acute tubular necrosis due to aortic cross clamping.

○ **What is the therapy of choice for a patient with chronic renal failure and pericarditis?**

Dialysis.

○   **What does acute renal failure in a patient with alcoholic cirrhosis and a urine sodium of less than 10 suggest?**

Pre-renal azotemia or hepatorenal syndrome.

○   **What does total and persistent anuria with renal failure suggest?**

Obstruction.

○   **Aminoglycosides are likely to cause what type of acute renal failure?**

Non-oliguric acute tubular necrosis (ATN).

○   **Anemia of chronic renal failure is likely to respond to what agent?**

Erythropoietin.

○   **What are the most common etiologies of chronic renal failure leading to dialysis in the U.S.?**

Hypertensive and diabetic renal disease.

○   **What are the first line oral phosphate binders used in CRF?**

Calcium carbonate and calcium acetate. Aluminum containing agents are best avoided.

○   **What co-morbid factors are likely to increase the risk of contrast induced ATN?**

Azotemia, diabetic nephropathy, CHF, multiple myeloma and dehydration.

○   **What are some long term complications seen with the use of aluminum containing phosphate binders?**

Aluminum induced osteomalacia, anemia and rarely dementia.

○   **What is the major therapy used to treat allergic interstitial nephritis not responding to discontinuation of the causative medication?**

Corticosteroids.

○   **What renal toxicity is seen with amphotericin B?**

Tubulointerstitial disease with a distal hypokalemic renal tubular acidosis and hypomagnesemia.

○   **What are the major complications seen after placement of percutaneous venous catheters for hemodialysis or CVVH?**

Bleeding, local infection and bacteremia. Pneumothorax and venous stenosis may occur with a subclavian catheter.

○   **What is the most common cause of acute renal failure?**

Acute tubular necrosis. This occurs after toxic or ischemic renal injuries.

O   **What clinical findings are seen with acute glomerulonephritis (GN)?**

1) Oliguria
2) Hypertension
3) Urine sediment containing RBCs, WBCs, protein and RBC casts
4) Edema

O   **What is the most common cause of post-infectious GN?**

Post streptococcal Group A beta-hemolytic glomerulonephritis. The GN is caused by immune complex deposition in glomeruli. Most patients completely recover normal renal function, spontaneously, within a few weeks.

O   **A urinalysis reveals RBC casts and dysmorphic RBCs. What is the probable origin of hematuria?**

Glomerulus.

O   **What are some common nephrotoxic agents?**

Aminoglycoside, NSAIDs, contrast dye and myoglobin.

O   **What is the definition of oliguria? Of anuria?**

Oliguria: Urine output < 500 ml/day
Anuria: Urine output < 100 ml/day

O   **What is the anatomical approach to ARF?**

Ask whether the site is pre-, intra-, or post-renal. Pre-renal is due to hypovolemia, intra-renal is mostly due to ATN or toxins and post-renal is due to obstruction.

O   **What is the most common cause of intrinsic (intra-) renal failure?**

Acute tubular necrosis (80 to 90%), resulting from an ischemic injury (the most common cause of ATN) or from a nephrotoxic agent. Less frequent causes of intrinsic renal failure (10 to 20%) include vasculitis, malignant hypertension, acute GN or allergic interstitial nephritis.

O   **If a urine dipstick is positive for blood, but a urine analysis is negative for RBCs, what is the probable disease?**

Rhabdomyolysis. Severe muscle damage results in free myoglobin in blood. Very high levels lead to acute renal failure.

O   **What two common medications can induce nephrogenic diabetes insipidus?**

Lithium and amphotericin B.

O   **What are some causes of false-positive hematuria?**

Food coloring, beets, paprika, rifampin, phenothiazines, Dilantin, myoglobin, or menstruation.

○   **What is the most common cause of hematuria?**

Lesions of the bladder or lower urinary tract. When hematuria originates in a kidney, the probable causes are polycystic kidney disease and nephropathy.

○   **What is the post void residual volume that suggests urinary retention?**

A volume greater than 60 cc.

○   **What is the most common origin of proteinuria?**

Pathology of the glomerulus. Other origins are tubular pathology or over production of protein.

○   **When is a post void residual urine considered abnormal?**

When it exceeds 200 mL.

○   **What bacteria is the most common cause of UTIs in uncatheterized elderly patients?**

E. coli.

○   **What is the number one cause of UTIs?**

E. coli. Other causative agents are also Gram-negative.

○   **What findings mark the presentation of a patient with rapidly progressive glomerulonephritis?**

Hematuria (most common), edema (periorbital), HTN, ascites, pleural effusion, rales, and anuria.

○   **A client in renal failure is prescribed polystyrene sulfonate (Kayexalate). What is the most likely reason for administering this drug?**

Elevated potassium levels.

○   **What is the physiological reason for Disequilibrium Syndrome?**

During dialysis, excess solutes are cleared from the blood at a faster pace than they can diffuse from the body's cells into the circulatory system.

○   **A patient in acute renal failure suddenly begins to have an increased urine output of 4-5 liters per day. What phase of acute renal failure is this called?**

The diuresis phase.

○   **A client complains of abdominal discomfort and has a palpable bladder, but is voiding only small amounts at request intervals. What would be the best nursing intervention?**

Obtain an order for urinary catheterization. The patient most likely has overflow retention of urine.

○   **In low doses, how does Dopamine affect the kidneys?**

It dilates the renal and mesenteric arteries increasing renal perfusion.

O   **What is a common and potentially dangerous complication of peritoneal dialysis?**

Peritonitis.

O   **What would be a priority nursing action if disequilibrium syndrome occurs during dialysis?**

Slow the rate of dialysis.

O   **What symptoms would a patient exhibit if disequilibrium syndrome was occurring during dialysis?**

Nausea, vomiting, headache, dizziness, seizures, and confusion.

O   **Where is the best place to secure a foley catheter to prevent irritation?**

To the inner thigh. The male patient may also have the foley secured to his abdomen.

O   **What serum blood test is the best indicator of renal function?**

Serum creatinine.

O   **What is the best way to obtain a urine specimen from a patient with a foley catheter?**

Clean the drainage tube collection site with betadine and aspirate urine from the drainage tube using a sterile needle.

O   **You are caring for a patient with chronic renal failure. You have been instructed not to take blood pressure in her right arm. What would be the reason for this?**

The patient most likely has an AV fistula or an external cannula in her right arm for dialysis. The blood pressure should never be taken in that arm because of the damage it could cause to the fistula.

O   **What is the medical goal of acute renal failure?**

Restore fluid and electrolyte balance so the body can achieve normal kidney function.

O   **What is the medical goal of chronic renal failure (CRF)?**

Maintain fluid and electrolyte balance artificially through dialysis for the remainder of the patient's life.

O   **What is the most common cause of cystitis?**

An infection introduced from the urethra.

O   **Is Milk of Magnesia an appropriate medication for patients with chronic renal failure? Why or why not?**

No. It can lead to magnesium toxicity since the kidneys are not able to excrete it.

O   **You insert a foley catheter into a patient with an overdistended bladder, but partially clamp the tubing to allow the urine to drain at a slow rate. Why?**

Rapidly emptying an overdistended bladder may cause shock and hypotension due to the rapid change in pressure in the abdominal viscera.

NEUROLOGY PEARLS

○ **A patient with closed head trauma has clear fluid leaking from his nares. How do you distinguish between excessive nasal secretions and a CSF leak?**

By checking the fluid for the presence of glucose. Glucose will be present in CSF but not nasal secretions.

○ **What is the mechanism for the development of a subdural empyema?**

Subdural empyemas occur most often as a sequelae of chronic sinusitis. There may be direct extension of bacterial pathogens from sinus cavities that are contiguous with the CNS or from septic venous thromboses. Subdural empyemas may also occur on first presentation or after several days of therapy in patients with bacterial meningitis

○ **What signs are associated with increased intracranial pressure?**

Headache, nausea, emesis, papilledema, systemic hypertension, bradycardia, irregular respiratory pattern and paralysis of upward gaze (setting sun sign).

○ **What is the treatment of choice for brain tumor edema?**

Dexamethasone.

○ **What is the most common cause of cerebrospinal fluid (CSF) leak?**

Basilar skull fractures.

○ **What measures assist in decreasing ICP?**

Elevation of the head of the bed to 30 degrees, intermittent drainage of CSF, hyperventilation and osmotic diuresis.

○ **What are the neurological signs of cerebellar abscesses?**

Horizontal nystagmus when looking towards the side of the lesion, ipsilateral dysmetria and ataxia.

○ **What are "pontine pupils?"**

Pinpoint but reactive pupils secondary to injury of the sympathetic fibers.

○ **What are the most common causes of worsened neurological deficit that occurs later in the course of traumatic spinal cord injury?**

Post-traumatic syrinx formation and persistent spinal cord compression.

○ **What percentage of patients with anterior cord syndromes regain the ability to walk without assistance?**

Fewer than 50%.

O   **T/F: Severe traumatic brain injury patients should be routinely hyperventilated.**

False.

O   **What are potential causes of delayed neurological deterioration in patients following intracranial aneurysm rupture?**

Bleeding, vasospasm, hydrocephalus and seizures.

O   **What are the major sources of brain abscesses?**

Direct extension from middle ear, mastoid and sinus infections, hematogenous spread and trauma.

O   **Bilateral facial paralysis associated with progressive ascending motor neuropathy of the lower extremities and elevated cerebrospinal fluid protein is characteristic of what clinical entity?**

Guillain-Barre syndrome.

O   **A patient is admitted to the critical care unit with the diagnosis of a subarachnoid hemorrhage secondary to an intracranial aneurysm. What complications may occur?**

More hemorrhage, hydrocephalus, seizure and cerebral vasospasm.

O   **What clinical findings occur in grade 4 subarachnoid hemorrhage?**

Stupor, hemiparesis and posturing.

O   **Why is there a higher incidence of complete neurologic loss with thoracic fractures than with cervical or lumbar fractures?**

The thoracic spinal canal has the least cross-sectional area for the spinal cord, thus allowing less room for movement of the cord. Furthermore, since the thoracic spine is so strong, a thoracic spine injury is the result of a tremendous force of injury. In addition, the blood supply to the thoracic cord has more of a watershed distribution than the other regions.

O   **What is cerebral perfusion pressure and what does it signify?**

CPP = MAP - ICP where MAP equals mean arterial pressure. CPP represents the pressure required to push blood from the arterial tree to the venous tree in the intracranial space.

O   **A multiple trauma patient is transferred to your facility with a history of head injury. The patient arrives intubated and sedated because he had a seizure prior to transport and was given 20 mg of IV diazepam. The patient now starts to seize again. What is the appropriate treatment?**

Phenytoin.

O   **A trauma patient is found to have a significant acute subdural hematoma by CT scan. What is the appropriate treatment?**

Emergency craniotomy.

O   **What is the etiology of vasospasm following subarachnoid hemorrhage?**

Contraction of the smooth muscle cells in the cerebral vasculature secondary to breakdown of red blood cells and release of hemoglobin into the CSF.

O   **What organisms are most commonly implicated in subdural empyemas?**

Staphylococci and *streptococci.*

O   **What is the mechanism of diffuse axonal injury?**

Rotation of the brain within the skull secondary to sudden deceleration.

O   **What is the earliest sign of central herniation?**

Decreased level of consciousness.

O   **What are the physical findings indicative of a basilar skull fracture?**

Periorbital and perimastoid ecchymosis. Patients may also suffer hearing loss, anosmia and CSF leaks.

O   **What is the most common source of bleeding from an epidural hematoma?**

Laceration of the middle meningeal artery.

O   **What is the source of bleeding from a subdural hematoma?**

Shearing of bridging veins between the dura and brain.

O   **What is the most common intracranial hemorrhage following head trauma?**

A subarachnoid hemorrhage.

O   **What are the most common forms of disturbed water balance after traumatic brain injury?**

Diabetes insipidus, the syndrome of inappropriate antidiuretic hormone (SIADH) and cerebral salt wasting.

O   **What are the characteristics of neurogenic pulmonary edema?**

Rapid onset of decreased lung compliance without elevation of the pulmonary capillary wedge pressure (PCWP), diffuse roentgenographic infiltrates and hypoxemia.

O   **What is the suspected mechanism of disseminated intravascular coagulation (DIC) associated with severe brain injury?**

Activation of the extrinsic clotting cascade by release of thromboplastin from the injured brain.

O   **What are the commonly employed surgical interventions for controlling medically refractory intracranial hypertension after trauma?**

Ventriculostomy drainage, hematoma evacuation, partial brain resection and decompressive craniectomy.

○   **What is the difference in pathogenesis and physiologic treatment of acute versus chronic subdural hematoma?**

An acute subdural hematoma occurs within 3 days of the incident, is the accumulation of blood in the subdural space that causes mass effect and requires a full craniotomy. A chronic subdural hematoma is usually older than 3 weeks and can often be adequately treated with a burr hole.

○   **A trauma patient presents with an altered level of consciousness, bilateral periorbital and perimastoid ecchymosis and hemotympanum. What injury do these signs suggest?**

A basilar skull fracture.

○   **What is the most significant indicator of poor outcome after head injury?**

Hypotension.

○   **What is the test of choice for a patient with a suspected subarachnoid hemorrhage?**

CT scan of the head. If CT is negative but suspicion is high, a spinal tap should be performed.

○   **What is the most important initial treatment for the severely head injured trauma patient?**

Establishing an airway.

○   **What is the classic presentation of an epidural hematoma?**

Brief loss of consciousness followed by a lucid interval with progressive loss of consciousness.

○   **What are the common locations for brain contusions?**

The frontal and temporal lobes.

○   **What is the prognosis for a patient recently diagnosed with amyotrophic lateral sclerosis (ALS)?**

Death 3 to 10 years after the onset of symptoms. ALS, also known as Lou Gehrig's disease, involves a progressive loss of the anterior horn cell function of the motor neurons. No sensory abnormalities are involved, just gradual weakness and atrophy of the muscles.

○   **Differentiate between decerebrate and decorticate posturing.**

Decerebrate posturing: elbows and legs extended (indicative of a midbrain lesion).
Decorticate posturing: elbows flexed and legs extended (suggesting a thalamic lesion).
Remember: DeCORticate = hands by the heart.

○   **What happens if light is directed into the eyes of a patient who is in a diabetic coma?**

The pupils will constrict.

○   **What is the most common cause of subarachnoid hemorrhage?**

Saccular aneurysm.

O   **What are other common causes of a subarachnoid hemorrhage?**

Rupture of cerebral artery aneurysm and arteriovenous malformation. These patients present with an abrupt, severe headache that can progress to syncope, nausea, vomiting, nuchal rigidity and non-focal neurological findings.

O   **Which is more common, subdural or epidural hemorrhaging?**

Subdural. Subdural hemorrhage results from tearing of the bridging veins. Bleeding occurs less rapidly because the veins, not arteries, are damaged.

O   **Differentiate between Korsakoff's psychosis and Wernicke's encephalopathy.**

Korsakoff's psychosis: Inability to process new information, i.e., to form new memories. This is a reversible condition resulting from brain damage induced by a thiamine deficiency that is secondary to chronic alcoholism.

Wernicke's encephalopathy: Also due to an alcohol induced thiamine deficiency. Patients experience decreased muscle coordination, ophthalmoplegia and confusion. The treatment is thiamine.

O   **How does bacterial meningitis differ from viral meningitis in terms of the corresponding CSF lab values?**

Bacterial meningitis is associated with low glucose and high protein levels, while viral meningitis will have normal glucose and normal protein levels.

O   **What is the most common medication associated with neuroleptic malignant syndrome?**

Haloperidol. Other drugs, especially antipsychotic medications, are also causative.

O   **What is the hallmark motor finding in neuroleptic malignant syndrome?**

"Lead pipe" rigidity.

O   **What is the significance of bilateral nystagmus with cold caloric testing?**

It signifies that an intact cortex and brainstem are present.

O   **Which are the two most common organisms to cause meningitis in patients with a ventriculo-peritoneal (VP) shunt?**

Staphylococcus epidermidis and Staphylococcus aureus.

O   **What potential adverse effect requires monitoring in patients treated with ticlopidine?**

Neutropenia.

O   **A head trauma patient develops hyponatremia. What criteria would diagnose SIADH?**

The criteria are: 1) Hyponatremia with a normal or mildly increased extracellular fluid volume, 2) elevated urinary osmolarity (>200 mOsm), 3) elevated urine sodium (>20 mEq/L), 4) no adrenal, thyroid or renal disease.

○   **What are the clinical features of myxedema coma?**

Non-pitting edema, hypothermia, bradycardia, dry skin and brittle hair.

○   **What are the neurological causes of diabetes insipidus?**

Lesions of the hypothalamus or pituitary caused by post-operative edema, head trauma, sarcoid, lymphoma, craniopharyngioma, pituitary adenoma and metastatic tumors.

○   **What are the clinical features of H. simplex encephalitis?**

Personality changes, fever, headache, delirium followed by coma, focal or generalized seizures, aphasia and focal motor symptoms.

○   **What drug is used to treat H. simplex encephalitis?**

Acyclovir.

○   **What drug will reduce the risk of vasospasm following subarachnoid hemorrhage?**

Nimodipine.

○   **What is the drug treatment for convulsive status epilepticus?**

Lorazepam followed by phenytoin are the initial drugs.

○   **What are the features of neuroleptic malignant syndrome?**

The features are altered mental status, fever, rigidity, irregular pulse, irregular blood pressure, tachycardia, diaphoresis and elevated CPK.

○   **What is the treatment for neuroleptic malignant syndrome?**

Immediate withdrawal of the neuroleptic drug. Sinemet, bromocriptine or dantrolene are used.

○   **What are the features of hypertensive encephalopathy?**

Diastolic blood pressure usually over 130 torr, papilledema and altered mental status.

○   **What are the earliest clinical features of uncal herniation?**

Uncal herniation begins with a unilateral enlarged pupil and a sluggish pupillary light reaction.

○   **What is the Cushing reflex?**

Elevation in blood pressure and reduction in pulse that follows an increase in intracranial pressure. It is a brainstem mediated reflex.

○   **What are the clinical criteria for the diagnosis of brain death?**

The criteria are: (1) coma is present from a known cause, (2) reversible causes of coma such as hypothermia (temperature < 32° C) or drug intoxication have been excluded and (3) there is no clinical evidence of brain or brainstem function.

O **Are there any predisposing factors to Guillain-Barre Syndrome (GBS)?**

Viral infection, gastrointestinal infection, immunization or surgery often precedes the neurological symptoms by 5 days to 3 weeks.

O **Can Guillain-Barre Syndrome (GBS) involve respiratory muscles quickly?**

Yes. It can start as rapidly progressing symmetric weakness, facial paresis, oropharyngeal and respiratory paresis, loss of DTRs and impaired sensation in the hands and feet.

O **When do GBS symptoms "level off"?**

After several days to three weeks.

O **Does early treatment with IVIG or plasmapheresis accelerate recovery in GBS?**

Yes. It also diminishes the incidence of long-term neurologic disability.

O **Can GBS be fatal?**

Yes. Especially with autonomic dysfunction, but very uncommonly.

O **What is the characteristic triad of normal pressure hydrocephalus?**

Dementia, incontinence and a gait apraxia (often described as a "magnetic" gait due to difficulty picking up the feet).

O **What is myasthenia gravis?**

Myasthenia gravis (MG) is an autoimmune disorder in which antibodies attack the postsynaptic end plate, resulting in focal (especially oculomotor) or generalized weakness that is worse after exercise. MG is associated with thymoma (15%) or thymic hypertrophy (50%) and most patients benefit from thymectomy. The diagnosis is aided by single fiber EMG studies, in which the pairing of muscle fiber action potentials show increased jitter (fluctuation in the timing of paired firing).

O **What are the essentials of the initial emergency management of seizures?**

As always, attend to the "ABCs" first. Spontaneous ventilation is absent during the tonic phase of a tonic-clonic seizure and is unpredictably present during the clonic phase. Anticonvulsant therapy may further impair central respiratory function.

O **What is the circulatory response to generalized seizure?**

There is usually striking sympathetic autonomic outflow with hypertension and tachycardia.

O **Do seizures cause brain injury?**

Evidence from animal studies suggests that generalized tonic-clonic seizures may cause irreversible neuronal damage. Less certain is the harm that may be caused by focal seizures. It is certainly safest to assume that generalized seizures lasting longer than 10 minutes may well have important adverse long term consequences for the patient and treat them aggressively.

○   **What is the initial therapy for seizures?**

The most popular initial therapy is diazepam. Lorazepam is also usually effective and provides a longer duration of anticonvulsant action. Both drugs may cause hypotension and respiratory depression.

○   **What is "status epilepticus"?**

Seizures continuing unabated for 15 to 30 minutes or more is a common operational definition of status epilepticus. Failure to return to a normal level of consciousness between episodic seizure activity over any period of time is also considered to be status epilepticus.

○   **What's the significance of status epilepticus?**

With status epilepticus, more significant complications become likely. These include hyperthermia from the muscle activity of the continuing seizure, metabolic acidosis and hypoxia and hypercarbia from respiratory compromise.

○   **What are the common causes of status epilepticus?**

Failure of patient with epilepsy to take medications
Meningitis
Hyponatremia and other metabolic abnormalities
Brain tumors
Stroke (infarct or hemorrhage)
Alcohol withdrawal

○   **What toxic ingestions are associated with seizures?**

Theophylline overdose causes CNS excitability and seizures. These seizures are usually focal rather than generalized. With acute ingestions, the seizures are usually brief and resolve spontaneously without medical intervention. Seizures occurring after chronic overdose may persist and not respond to usual drug interventions.

Hemodialysis or charcoal hemoperfusion is an option in patients with status epilepticus associated with high blood levels of aminophylline.

Tricyclic antidepressant overdosage is associated with seizures. These may be myoclonic jerks or generalized convulsions. Impaired level of consciousness is typically associated with blood levels of tricyclics high enough to cause seizures.

Lidocaine, cocaine and other local anesthetics can also produce seizures. These are usually of brief duration and self-limited. When they are not, the usual supportive care and conventional anticonvulsant therapy can be expected to produce satisfactory outcomes.

Isoniazid seizures are characterized by intractability to the usual anti-seizure medications. Pyridoxine is the drug of choice.

○   **A 52 year old known alcoholic male presents to the emergency department with repeated seizures. What is the differential diagnosis?**

It is the same as for any other patient. Alcohol ingestion per se is not thought to promote seizures. Withdrawal from alcohol can produce seizures ("rum fits") from 8 to 48 hours after cessation of or decreasing the rate of alcohol intake. Seizures associated with alcohol withdrawal usually are brief generalized tonic-clonic and limited to a single episode. Less commonly, status epilepticus occurs in alcohol withdrawal. Many alcoholics with seizures have an underlying structural (traumatic) basis for their seizures.

Extraordinary alcohol ingestion can be associated with hypoglycemia, which can be severe enough to cause seizures.

O   **Describe the symptoms and signs of myasthenia gravis.**

Weakness and fatigability with ptosis, diplopia and blurred vision are the initial symptoms most patients. Bulbar muscle weakness is also common with dysarthria and dysphagia.

O   **Under what conditions does neurogenic pulmonary edema occur?**

Neurogenic pulmonary edema is commonly associated with increased intracranial pressure. It is commonly seen with head trauma, subarachnoid hemorrhage and seizures.

O   **How many minutes of cerebral anoxia will result in irreversible brain injury?**

Over 8 minutes.

O   **What is the BEST indication for assisted ventilation in a 70 kg patient with Guillian-Barre syndrome?**

Abnormal blood gases are a late finding in patients with GBS or other neuromuscular syndromes and bedside pulmonary functions including forced vital capacity (FVC) are the most sensitive.

O   **What is the gold standard for monitoring ICP?**

Ventricular catheter.

O   **A patient opens his eyes to voice, makes incomprehensible sounds, and withdraws to painful stimulus. What is his GCS?**

9.

O   **Define the properties of the Glasgow Coma Scale.**

Eye opening	Verbal activity	Motor activity
4. Spontaneous	5. Oriented	6. Obeys command
3. To command	4. Confused	5. Localizes pain
2. To pain	3. Inappropriate	4. Withdraws to pain
1. None	2. Incomprehensible	3. Flexion to pain
	1. None	2. Extension to pain
		1. None

O   **What are the signs and symptoms of phenytoin toxicity?**

Seizure, heart blocks, bradyarrhythmias, hypotension, and coma. All dangerous cardiovascular complications of phenytoin overdose result from parenteral administration. High levels after PO doses do not cause such signs in a stable patient.

○   **Differentiate between dementia and delirium.**

Dementia - Irreversible impaired functioning secondary to changes/deficits in memory, spatial concepts, personality, cognition, language, motor and sensory skills, judgment, or behavior. There is no change in consciousness.

Delirium - A reversible organic mental syndrome reflecting deficits in attention, organized thinking, orientation, speech, memory, and perception. Patients are frequently confused, anxious, excited, and have hallucinations. A change in consciousness can be observed.

○   **Describe the signs and symptoms of spinal shock.**

Spinal shock represents complete loss of spinal cord function below the level of injury. Patients have flaccid paralysis, complete sensory loss, areflexia, and loss of autonomic function. Such patients are usually bradycardic, hypotensive, hypothermic, and vasodilated.

○   **What symptoms are expected with a phenytoin level of > 20, > 30, and > 40 g/ml?**

> 20: lateral gaze nystagmus.
> 30: lateral gaze nystagmus plus increased vertical nystagmus with upward gaze.
> 40: lethargy, confusion, dysarthria, and psychosis.

○   **Why would you be concerned if a quadriplegic suddenly develops a severe headache?**

It is a symptom of autonomic dysreflexia. Bladder distention is one of the most common causes.

○   **When monitoring a client following a CVA, what changes in vital signs should be reported to the MD immediately?**

Increased blood pressure, decreased pulse, and decreased respiratory rate.

○   **What is the basic principle of bladder training for the quadriplegic?**

Setting up a schedule where the patient empties his bladder at the same time every day.

○   **Why is mannitol given in the treatment of head injuries?**

It is a powerful diuretic that will help reduce cerebral edema.

○   **What does the term "stroke in evolution" mean?**

A stroke in which neurologic changes continue to occur for 24 to 48 hours after the initial incident.

○   **What are the first four things you should do if a patient is having a grand mal seizure?**

Ease the patient to the floor, protect the head, protect him/her from injury, and maintain a patent airway.

○   **Why should a patient who is having a seizure not be restrained?**

Strong muscle contractions could cause the patient to injure himself.

O   **What behavior would you expect from a patient following a seizure?**

The patient is usually disoriented and tired (post-ictal), sleeping for a long period of time.

O   **What respiratory pattern is indicative of increased intercranial pressure?**

Slow, irregular respirations.

O   **What should be your main focus when a patient is having a seizure?**

Maintaining an open airway.

O   **How long can spinal shock last following a spinal cord injury?**

It can last for several weeks after the initial injury.

O   **What is the most serious complication in a patient who has had an acute stroke?**

Increasing ICP.

O   **What is an indication that spinal shock is resolving?**

The return of reflex activity in the legs and arms below the level of the injury.

O   **What is a positive Babinski reflex?**

Toe fanning when the sole is stroked from heel to toe.

O   **What are some of the symptoms of hypertensive encephalopathy?**

Elevated blood pressure, hemiparesis, loss of vision, disorientation, and seizures.

O   **Why is a nasogastric tube inserted when a client has severe head trauma?**

To decompress the stomach and prevent aspiration. The risk of aspiration is greater in an unconscious client.

O   **What is the purpose of mannitol in treating head trauma?**

It is an osmotic diuretic used to decrease intercranial pressure caused by cerebral edema.

O   **What side-effect can occur from rapidly infusing phenytoin sodium (Dilantin)?**

Cardiotoxicity leading to bradycardia, hypotension, cardiac arrest, and asystole.

O   **Why would the Trendelenburg position be contraindicated after brain tumor removal?**

This could cause an increase in intercranial pressure.

INFECTIOUS DISEASE PEARLS

○ **What is the most common complication of AIDS?**

Pneumocystis carinii pneumonia (PCP). Kaposi's sarcoma is the second most common.

○ **What organisms are most commonly responsible for overwhelming postsplenectomy sepsis?**

Pneumococci, meningococci, *E. coli*, *H. influenzae*, staphylococci and streptococci.

○ **Describe the skin lesions associated with a Pseudomonas aeruginosa infection.**

Pale, erythematous lesions, 1 cm in size, with an ulcerated necrotic center.

○ **The initial therapy for PCP includes which antibiotics?**

Trimethoprim-sulfamethoxazole (preferred) or pentamidine.

○ **What other medication should be prescribed to a patient with PCP?**

Corticosteroids.

○ **What is the definition of nosocomial pneumonia?**

Pneumonia occurring in patients who have been hospitalized for at least 72 hours.

○ **What is the single most important risk factor for hospital acquired bacterial pneumonia?**

Endotracheal intubation.

○ **Among patients with cystic fibrosis, what bacteria are seen with increased frequency as causes of pneumonia?**

Pseudomonas aeruginosa and *Staphylococcus aureus*.

○ **What ubiquitous protozoan is responsible for a diffuse interstitial pneumonitis in immunocompromised patients?**

Pneumocystis carinii.

○ **What is the most common source of gram-negative infections in patients with septic shock?**

The urinary tract.

○ **What antibiotic has been consistently effective against penicillin resistant *Streptococcus pneumoniae*?**

Vancomycin.

○   **What are the two most important risk factors for the development of anaerobic lung abscess?**

Poor oral hygiene and a predisposition toward aspiration.

○   **What are the two most important routes of transmission of nosocomial bacterial pneumonia?**

Person-to-person transmission via healthcare workers and contaminated ventilator tubing.

○   **How may stress ulcer prophylaxis in ICU patients contribute to the development of nosocomial pneumonia?**

By raising the gastric pH and increasing bacterial colonization.

○   **What is the commonest cause of meningitis in HIV disease?**

Cryptococcus.

○   **What is the significance of a patient who received amphotericin bladder irrigation and has not cleared their urine of candida?**

Patients who do not clear the yeast from the urine should be evaluated for urinary tract obstruction with a renal ultrasound. Candidal urine casts are a sign of upper urinary tract involvement. Patients who have infection of the upper tract will require treatment with amphotericin. A patient who is clinically deteriorating and at high risk for systemic infection, such as the neutropenic patient, should be evaluated for the possibility of disseminated candidiasis.

○   **What is the epidemiology of necrotizing fasciitis?**

Necrotizing fasciitis is a severe infection distinguished by necrosis of the fascia and subcutaneous tissues, resulting in undermining of the skin. Onset is abrupt and is more common in diabetics, alcoholics and IV drug abusers, usually precipitated by a traumatized area of skin.

○   **What are the clinical findings of necrotizing fasciitis?**

Initial physical findings may mimic cellulitis with swollen, very tender, erythematous skin. Unlike cellulitis, the margins are usually not well demarcated and the involved area typically becomes anesthetic due to the destruction of cutaneous nerves by the inflammatory process. Some patients develop subcutaneous gas and grossly necrotic skin or bulla formation. Very high fever and signs of toxicity disproportionate to the physical findings suggest necrotizing fasciitis. The superficial skin findings can be thought of as the tip of the iceberg.

○   **What is the treatment for necrotizing fasciitis?**

Intravenous penicillin/clindamycin/gentamicin, and assertive surgical debridement are both necessary.

○   **What patients are at increased risk for developing sternal wound infections and mediastinitis after cardiac surgery?**

Sternal wound infections occur with an incidence of 1 to 5% after median sternotomy. Patients at increased risk include diabetics, those with bilateral inferior mammary takedowns, re-operations and patients with a low cardiac output state. Responsible microorganisms are predominately *Staphylococcus aureus*, *Staphylococcus epidermidis*, *pseudomonas* species and *enterobacteriaceae*.

○   **What are the clinical features in a patient with such an infection?**

Symptoms manifest a week or more post-operatively and include fever, drainage, inability to wean from mechanical ventilation and an unstable sternum. More catastrophic complications related to sternal wound infection include hemorrhage from the heart and great vessels. This may occur by several mechanisms, including right ventricular rupture, suture line leaks at the aortotomy site and vein graft anastomotic leaks.

○   **How are sternal wound infections managed?**

Sternal wound infections are commonly managed with operative debridement and muscle flaps. Other methods including a "double-catheter irrigation technique" are under evaluation.

○   **What side effects have been associated with the use of vancomycin?**

Red man syndrome, characterized by flushing of the face, thorax and hypotension, is caused by histamine release and is associated with rapid infusion. It is not considered to be an allergic reaction. Ototoxicity and nephrotoxicity may occur, especially with older preparations of the drug.

○   **How are prosthetic valve infections classified?**

Prosthetic valve infections are classified as early (< 2 months post-operative) and late (>2 months post-operative). Both types are very serious infections, although early valve infections tend to have a worse prognosis. Bacteremic patients with new prosthetic valves should be suspected to have endocarditis.

○   **When do patients with prosthetic valve infections require surgery?**

If annular involvement becomes apparent, the patient requires operative debridement and valve replacement. Antibiotic therapy alone may be curative in cases of late bioprosthetic endocarditis, which is usually valvular in nature. However, many patients require surgery due to serious valvular dysfunction or bulky vegetations. Mechanical valve infections are also around the suture ring. Patients presenting in shock or severe congestive heart failure require emergent surgery.

○   **What time after insertion are pulmonary artery catheters considered at high risk to be infected?**

After 72 hours.

○   **What are the most common organisms involved with line infections?**

Staphylococcus epidermidis and *Staphylococcus aureus*.

○   **How does a subphrenic abscess present?**

It follows surgery for a ruptured viscus, cholecystitis or penetrating abdominal wound. Patients may complain of right upper quadrant or shoulder pain in addition to fever and chills. Subphrenic abscesses occur far more commonly on the right. The chest x-ray typically reveals an elevated hemidiaphragm and may show a pleural effusion or an air/fluid level below the diaphragm in more advanced cases. CT is diagnostic.

○   **What adverse reactions may be seen with amphotericin infusion?**

Release of tumor necrosis factor has been postulated to cause the fever, rigors and a drop in blood pressure commonly seen with administration of Amphotericin B. Hypotension occurs frequently in debilitated patients, especially in the early stages of treatment. This is the reason why a 1mg test dose is given prior to a full daily treatment dose. True allergic reactions to Amphotericin B are uncommon.

O   **What is streptococcal toxic shock syndrome?**

The recent emergence of highly virulent strains of Group A Streptococcus pyogenes has been associated with severe invasive disease that may cause multiorgan failure. This fulminant process may be precipitated by seemingly minor trauma to skin or mucosal surfaces and is rarely associated with streptococcal pharyngitis. Exotoxin production by these strains has been implicated as the cause of tissue injury, which often includes organ failure, ARDS and necrotizing fasciitis. Patients with prior exposure to streptococcal M proteins are relatively protected from this syndrome.

A definite case includes isolation of group A streptococci from a normally <u>sterile</u> site (e.g., blood, CSF, pleural or peritoneal fluid) and the presence of hypotension or shock plus at least two of the following signs: renal impairment, disseminated intravascular coagulation, abnormal liver function, ARDS, erythematous rash with or without desquamation and soft tissue necrosis (e.g., necrotizing fasciitis, myositis or gangrene).

A probable case has group A streptococcus isolated from a normally <u>nonsterile</u> site (eg, pharynx, skin and sputum), in addition to hypotension, shock and at least two of the above listed signs.

O   **What are risk factors for developing sinusitis in the intensive care unit?**

Nasally intubated patients develop sinusitis with an incidence from 2 to 25%. This complication is related to trauma, edema and obstruction of drainage from the ostia in the lateral nasal wall. Trauma patients with facial fractures, patients with limited head mobility and those who require nasal packing and nasogastric tubes are especially prone.

O   **What is the clinical scenario in which sinusitis occurs in the ICU?**

Though sinusitis develops relatively early after nasal intubation, the diagnosis may not be readily apparent, as it is often not accompanied by purulent nasal drainage. Most typically patients present with fever and leukocytosis and may progress to sepsis.

O   **How is sinusitis that occurs in the ICU diagnosed and treated?**

Sinus CT scans will confirm the diagnosis, but antral taps for gram stain and culture are recommended to guide treatment. Unlike community acquired sinusitis, *Staphylococcus aureus* and gram negative rods are the most common organisms. Polymicrobial infections are frequently seen. Removal of any foreign body is necessary. Phenylephrine nasal drops decrease edema and promote drainage. Some patients require repeated antral lavage. Patients who are nasotracheally intubated should be reintubated orally.

O   **What are the characteristics of drug fever?**

Patients with a drug related fever often will appear relatively well, despite a high temperature. Usual temperatures are in the range of 102 to 104 degrees Fahrenheit, though low grade and extreme elevations may also be seen. Sustained fevers and a relative bradycardia are typical. Besides antibiotics, other common causes of drug fever include amphotericin, procainamide, salicylates, barbiturates, phenytoin, quinidine and interferon. Drug fever is not always accompanied by rash.

O   **What are the risk factors for developing primary peritonitis?**

Primary peritonitis, also known as spontaneous bacterial peritonitis, is an acute or subacute bacterial infection of the peritoneum unrelated to the usual causes of peritonitis, such as a perforated viscus or intra-abdominal abscess. The vast majority of cases occur in patients with alcoholic cirrhosis, but patients with cirrhosis and ascites from other causes are also predisposed.

O   **What are the clinical findings and treatment for primary peritonitis?**

Fever and abdominal pain are present in most patients, but peritoneal signs may not be appreciable. The most useful findings on analysis of peritoneal fluid include an elevated white blood cell count. Gram stains of peritoneal fluid are negative in the majority of cases, so empiric treatment should be initiated if there is suspicion. These infections tend to be due to a single organism in most cases, commonly *Escherichia coli* and *Streptococcus pneumoniae*, unlike secondary peritonitis which is usually polymicrobial.

O   **Which antibiotics are most frequently implicated as precipitants for Stevens-Johnson syndrome?**

Stevens-Johnson syndrome or erythema multiforme major, is a serious hypersensitivity reaction that presents with a generalized vesiculobullous eruption of the skin, mouth, eyes and genitals. Many drugs have been identified as triggering this reaction, but the most common antibiotics are the sulfa drugs and the penicillins. Stevens-Johnson syndrome has also been seen in patients with recent mycoplasma infections.

O   **What causes toxic shock syndrome (TSS)?**

An exotoxin derived from certain strains of Staphylococcus aureus. Other organisms that cause toxic shock syndrome are group A streptococci, Pseudomonas aeruginosa and Streptococcus pneumoniae. Tampons, IUD's, septic abortions, sponges, soft tissue abscesses, osteomyelitis, nasal packing and postpartum infections all can house these organisms.

O   **What dermatological changes occur with TSS?**

Initially, the patient will have a blanching erythematous rash that lasts for 3 days. After 10 days there will be a desquamation of the palms and soles.

O   **What are the criteria for the diagnosis of TSS?**

All of the following must be present: T > 38.9° C (102° F), rash, systolic BP < 90 orthostasis, involvement of 3 or more organ systems (GI, renal, musculoskeletal, mucosal, hepatic, hematologic or CNS) and negative serologic tests for diseases such as RMSF, hepatitis B, measles, leptospirosis and syphilis.

O   **How should a patient with TSS be treated?**

Fluids, vasopressor support, vaginal irrigation with iodine or saline and anti-staphylococcal penicillin or cephalosporin with anti-beta-lactamase activity. Rifampin should be considered to eliminate the carrier state.

O   **What is the most common oral manifestation of AIDS?**

Oropharyngeal thrush. Other AIDS-related oropharyngeal diseases include Kaposi's sarcoma, hairy leukoplakia, and non-Hodgkin's lymphoma.

O   **Describe the pathophysiologic features of HIV.**

HIV attacks the T4 helper cells. The genetic material of HIV consists of singlestranded RNA. HIV has been found in semen, vaginal secretions, blood and blood products, saliva, urine, cerebrospinal fluid, tears, alveolar fluid, synovial fluid, breast milk, transplanted tissue, and amniotic fluid. There has not been documentation of infection from casual contact.

❍   **Name the most common causes of fever in HIV-infected patients.**

HIV related fever, Mycobacterium aviumintracellular, CMV, and non-Hodgkin's and Hodgkin's lymphoma.

❍   **What is the most common cause of focal encephalitis in AIDS patients?**

Toxoplasmosis. Symptoms include focal neurologic deficits, headache, fever, altered mental status, and seizures. Ring enhancing lesions are evident on CT.

❍   **What is the risk of contracting HIV infection after an occupational exposure?**

0.32% for needle sticks and 0.08% for mucus membrane exposure to high risk body fluids. Eighty percent of the occupational exposure-related infections are from needle sticks.

❍   **What bacteria is the most common cause of UTIs in uncatheterized elderly patients?**

E. coli.

❍   **What is the most common source of sepsis in the elderly?**

Respiratory > Urinary > Intra-abdominal.

❍   **What are the classic signs and symptoms of TB?**

Night sweats, fever, weight loss, malaise, cough, and a green/yellow sputum which most commonly is seen in the mornings.

❍   **Who should receive prophylaxis after exposure to Neisseria meningitidis?**

People living with the patient or having close intimate contact.

❍   **You note that a patient's WBC is below 1,000 mm³. What special interventions would be called for?**

Reverse isolation precautions to decrease any risk of opportunistic infection.

❍   **A client is being admitted for bacterial meningitis. What type of room would be the most appropriate?**

A private room to reduce the spread of the infection.

❍   **A client is admitted with pneumonia and the MD orders sputum cultures to be obtained before antibiotics are begun. The patient is unable to cough up any sputum. What should you do?**

Obtain an order to have a sputum sample induced with an aerosol treatment. If still unsuccessful, notify the MD.

○ **What is the mode of transmission for the tubercle bacillus?**

Inhalation of tubercle-laden droplets.

○ **What type of lab study is used to determine if the tubercle bacilli is present in sputum?**

Acid-fast staining.

○ **What age groups are at risk for septic shock due to infection?**

The very young and the elderly.

○ **What is the purpose of administering zidovudine (Retrovir, AZT) to a patient?**

It interferes with the replication of the HIV virus in hopes of slowing the conversion of HIV to AIDS.

○ **What would you most likely find upon assessment of a patient with epididymitis?**

Scrotal swelling and severe tenderness.

○ **A urinalysis report indicates the presence of red blood cells and white blood cells. What is the most likely cause?**

Urinary tract infection.

○ **What are the first four things you should do if a patient is having a grand mal seizure?**

Ease the patient to the floor, protect the head, protect him/her from injury, and maintain a patent airway.

○ **What type of infection is produced by clostridium perfringens?**

Gas gangrene.

○ **When performing pin care, should you remove the crusting or scab formation that develops around the pin or should it be left and treated as a wound which is healing?**

Remove the scab formation. It can trap bacteria causing an infection to develop.

○ **In a postoperative patient, what organism is most likely to cause septicemia?**

E. coli.

○ **What are the signs and symptoms of septicemia?**

Fever, chills, rash, abdominal distension, prostration, pain, headache, nausea, and diarrhea.

○ **What are the early indications of gangrene?**

Edema, pain, redness, tissue darkening, and coldness in the affected body part.

○ **What are the complications associated with aminoglycoside use?**

Nephrotoxicity and ototoxicity.

○   **Aminoglycoside antibiotics infused too rapidly can cause what side effect?**

Hypotension.

HEMATOLOGY
AND ONCOLOGY PEARLS

○ **What are the pulmonary manifestations of sickle cell disease?**

Acute chest syndrome, bacterial pneumonia, cor pulmonale, reduction in DLCO, reduced static lung volumes and a right shifted oxygen dissociation curve.

○ **What is the mechanism for the acute chest syndrome?**

Microvascular occlusion by sickle cells which ultimately results in alveolar wall destruction and subsequent fibrosis.

○ **What is the treatment for a severe case of acute chest syndrome?**

Exchange transfusion.

○ **What are the common pathogens causing pneumonia in sickle cell patients?**

S. pneumoniae, *H. influenzae*, alpha-hemolytic streptococcus and salmonella.

○ **What is the hyperleukocytosis syndrome?**

Vascular occlusion due to high numbers of circulating leukemic cells. Pulmonary manifestations include hypoxemia, dyspnea, infiltrates and fever in the absence of infection. The treatment is emergent leukapheresis.

○ **What is the acute chest syndrome in sickle cell lung disease?**

Fever, chest pain, leukocytosis and pulmonary infiltrates. The major dilemma is in distinguishing infarction from pneumonia. Fat embolism is a less common cause.

○ **A SICU trauma patient is noted to be oozing from multiple wound sites. What tests and accompanying results would be consistent with disseminated intravascular coagulopathy (DIC)?**

Decreased platelet count, elevated prothrombin time, elevated activated partial thromboplastin time, decreased fibrinogen, elevated fibrin degradation products and presence of D-dimers.

○ **It is generally agreed that most patients with active bleeding and platelet counts < 50,000/mm^3 should receive platelet transfusion. How much will the platelet count be raised for each unit of platelets infused?**

5,000 to 10,000/mm^3.

○ **What five treatments are available to bleeding patients with liver disease?**

1) Transfusion with RBCs (maintains hemodynamic stability)
2) Vitamin K
3) Fresh frozen plasma
4) Platelet transfusion
5) DDAVP (Desmopressin)

○   **What are the clinical complications of DIC?**

Bleeding, thrombosis and purpura fulminans.

○   **Which laboratory studies are most helpful in diagnosing DIC?**

1) PT and PTT (prolonged)
2) Platelet count (usually low)
3) Fibrinogen level (low)
4) Presence of D-dimers

○   **What are the most common hemostatic abnormalities in patients infected with HIV?**

Thrombocytopenia and acquired circulating anticoagulants (causes prolongation of aPTT).

○   **Which clinical crises are seen in patients with sickle-cell disease?**

1) Vasoocclusive (thrombotic)
2) Hematologic (sequestration and aplastic)
3) Infectious

○   **Which is the most common type of sickle-cell crisis?**

Vaso-occlusive.

○   **How much will the infusion of 1 unit of RBCs raise the hemoglobin and hematocrit in a 70-kg patient?**

Hemoglobin: 1 g/dl. Hematocrit: 3%.

○   **What is the first step in treating all immediate transfusion reactions?**

Stop the transfusion.

○   **What is the current recommended emergency replacement therapy for massive hemorrhage?**

Type-specific, uncrossmatched blood. Type O negative, which may be immediately life saving in certain situations, carries the risk of life threatening transfusion reactions.

○   **What is the only crystalloid fluid compatible with RBCs?**

Normal saline.

○   **What are the major causes of GI bleeding in cancer patients?**

Hemorrhagic gastritis and peptic ulcer disease.

○   **What is appropriate initial treatment for a life threatening level of hypercalcemia of 16 mg per deciliter?**

0.9 NS at 5 to 10 liters per day. After attaining euvolemia, furosemide can be given. Additional therapy includes pamidronate, glucocorticoids, mithramycin or calcitonin.

○   **What blood product is given when the coagulation abnormality is unknown?**

Fresh frozen plasma.

○   **What is the most important aspect of treating DIC?**

Correcting the underlying disorder (usually septic shock).

○   **What are the signs and symptoms of splenic sequestration crisis?**

Pallor, weakness, lethargy, disorientation, shock, decreased level of consciousness and enlarged spleen.

○   **What is the treatment of splenic sequestration crisis?**

Rapid infusion of saline and transfusion of red cells.

○   **What is the predominant symptom in DIC?**

Bleeding.

○   **What are some common ischemic complications of DIC?**

Renal failure, seizures, coma, pulmonary infarction and hemorrhagic necrosis of the skin.

○   **What are the common lab findings in DIC?**

Decreased platelets, increased PT and PTT, decreased fibrinogen, increased FDP and D-dimers.

○   **What causes febrile reactions to blood and what is the incidence?**

The febrile reaction is the most common mild transfusion reaction and occurs in 0.5% to 4% of transfusions. It is caused by donor antibodies to antigens on the recipient's WBCs.

○   **What is transfusion related acute lung injury?**

It is a form of noncardiogenic pulmonary edema, occurring within 2 to 4 hours after a transfusion. This reaction should be suspected in any patient who develops pulmonary edema after a transfusion in which volume overload is thought to be unlikely. Clinical signs of respiratory distress vary from mild dyspnea to severe hypoxia. It usually resolves within 48 hours in response to oxygen, mechanical ventilation and other forms of supportive treatments.

○   **A patient on chemotherapy for his Burkitt's lymphoma is found to be hyperkalemic, hypocalcemic, hyperphosphatemic and hyperuracemic. What is the presumptive diagnosis?**

Tumor lysis syndrome.

○   **Which solutions are considered incompatible with PRBC?**

Calcium containing solutions should not be added to blood, particularly at slow infusion rates, because small clots may form due to the presence of calcium in excess of the chelating ability of the citrate anticoagulant.

○   **What are the problems associated with citrate in a massive transfusion?**

Massive transfusions increase citrate levels and decrease ionized calcium levels.

○   **Which drug most commonly causes true allergic reactions?**

Penicillin, which accounts for approximately 90% of all true allergic reactions. 95% of fatal anaphylactic reactions are caused by penicillin. Parenterally administered penicillin is more than twice as likely to cause a fatal anaphylactic reaction than the orally administered type.

○   **What is the treatment of choice for patients in anaphylactic shock?**

Epinephrine, 0.3-0.5 mg intravenously. If there is no IV access, inject the medication into the venous plexus at the base of the tongue.

○   **Which types of blood loss are indicative of a bleeding disorder?**

Spontaneous bleeding from many sites, bleeding from non-traumatic sites, delayed bleeding several hours after trauma, and bleeding into deep tissues or joints.

○   **What common drugs have been implicated in predisposing to acquired bleeding disorders?**

Ethanol, salicylates, NSAIDs, warfarin, and antibiotics.

○   **Below what platelet count is spontaneous hemorrhage likely to occur?**

< 10,000/mm^3.

○   **How can an overdose of warfarin be treated? What are the advantages and disadvantages of each treatment?**

Treatment depends on the severity of symptoms, not the degree of prolongation of the prothrombin time (PT). If there are no signs of bleeding, temporary discontinuation may be all that is necessary; if bleeding is present, treatment can be initiated with fresh frozen plasma (FFP) or Vitamin K.

Advantages of FFP: rapid repletion of coagulation factors and control of hemorrhage. Disadvantages: volume overload, possible viral transmission

Advantages of Vitamin K: ease of administration. Disadvantages: possible anaphylaxis when given IV; delayed onset of 12-24 hours; effects may last up to 2 weeks, making anticoagulation of the patient difficult or impossible.

○   **What three laboratory studies would be most helpful in establishing the diagnosis of DIC?**

1) Prothrombin time—prolonged.
2) Platelet count—usually low.
3) Fibrinogen level—low.

○ **What are the most common hemostatic abnormalities in patients infected with HIV?**

Thrombocytopenia and acquired circulating anticoagulants (causes prolongation of the PTT).

○ **What is the leading cause of death in hemophiliacs?**

AIDS.

○ **What are the three conditions under which the transfusion of PRBC's should be considered?**

1) Acute hemorrhage (blood loss > 1,500 ml).
2) Surgical blood loss > 2 L.
3) Chronic anemia (Hgb < 7–8 g/dL, symptomatic, or with underlying cardiopulmonary disease).

○ **What factors indicate the need for typing and cross-matching of blood in an emergency setting?**

1) Evidence of shock from whatever cause.
2) Known blood loss > 1,000 ml.
3) Gross GI bleeding.
4) Hgb < 10; Hct < 30.
5) Potential of going to surgery with further significant blood loss.

○ **What infection carries the highest risk of transmission by blood transfusion?**

Hepatitis C.

○ **What electrolyte abnormality is commonly associated with the transfusion of packed red blood cells?**

Hypocalcemia secondary to citrate toxicity. Citrate, when rapidly infused, binds ionized calcium and therefore decreases the calcium level. Hyperkalemia may also develop with rapidly packed red blood cell transfusion, especially if the patient is in renal failure or if the blood products are old.

○ **What is the universal donor blood?**

Type Rh negative blood, type O.

○ **What are the common presentations of a transfusion reaction?**

Myalgia, dyspnea, fever associated with hypocalcemia, hemolysis, allergic reactions, hyperkalemia, citrate toxicity, hypothermia, coagulopathies, and altered hemoglobin function.

○ **What is the most common transfusion reaction?**

Fever.

○ **You note that a patient's WBC is below 1,000 mm^3. What special interventions would be called for?**

Reverse isolation precautions to decrease any risk of opportunistic infection.

○   **You are ordered to start an IV on a client with a low platelet count. What special precautions should you take?**

Hold pressure on all unsuccessful venipuncture sites for 10 minutes, use a small gauge IV catheter, wrap the area with gauze to preserve skin integrity, and observe for any bleeding around the puncture site.

○   **An MD orders streptokinase for treatment of an MI. What is the most harmful complication of this medication that you should assess for?**

Bleeding.

○   **Approximately how many milliliters of fluid are in one unit of packed red blood cells?**

250.

○   **Following heart surgery, your client experiences persistent bleeding from the incision site. What drug will the physician most likely order to help stop this bleeding?**

Protamine sulfate.

○   **When administering blood to a client, what type of reaction should you always assess for?**

Anaphylaxis, hemolytic transfusion reactions, bacteremia, and fluid overload.

○   **Which lab test is used to determining the dosage of warfarin (Coumadin)?**

PT prothrombin time.

○   **A patient on a heparin drip is to be switched to oral warfarin (Coumadin). The physician orders warfarin (Coumadin) therapy to begin 36 hours before the heparin is discontinued. Why?**

It takes 36-72 hours for Coumadin to take effect.

○   **Why would a patient with a common bile duct obstruction be monitored for prolonged bleeding?**

Because if bleeding is present, bile is prevented from entering the intestinal tract, thus preventing the absorption of fat soluble vitamins such as vitamin K, which is necessary for prothrombin formation.

○   **When administering blood, what solution should be administered along with the blood in a tandem set-up?**

Normal saline.

○   **Describe petechia.**

Tiny, round, purplish-red spots that appear on the skin and mucous membranes as a result of intradermal or submucosal hemorrhage.

○   **What is purpura?**

Any purple skin discoloration caused by blood extravasation.

ELECTROLYTE, ACID-BASE AND ENDOCRINE PEARLS

○ **What is the relationship between serum sodium to water balance?**

Generally, due to renal mechanisms:
Hypernatremia means "too little free water", rather than "too much sodium."
Hyponatremia means "too much free water", rather than "too little sodium."

○ **How is plasma sodium interpreted in the presence of hyperglycemia?**

High glucose concentration draws water out of cells and dilutes sodium in plasma.
For every 100 mg/dl of glucose above 200 mg/dl the serum sodium is decreased by 1.6 mEq/L.

○ **What are the symptoms of hyponatremia? At what sodium levels do they present?**

Acute decrease in plasma sodium produces lethargy, nausea, headaches, confusion, weakness, abdominal cramps, vomiting, delirium, seizures and coma. Acutely serum sodium has to drop to around 125 mEq/L for symptoms to be present.

Coma and seizures are seen at sodium levels below 115 mEq/L.
Chronic hyponatremia may be asymptomatic until sodium drops below 115 mEq/L.

○ **How fast should hyponatremia be corrected?**

No faster than 0.5 to 1.0 mEq/L/hour of sodium. The initial goal is to correct to sodium level no higher than 120 to 125 mEq/L

○ **What is the complication if hyponatremia is corrected too rapidly?**

Central pontine myelinolysis or osmotic demyelinating syndrome. This syndrome can present several days after the treatment of hyponatremia. Symptoms include quadraparesis with swallowing dysfunction, pseudobulbar palsy and inability to speak.

○ **Loss of free water can cause hypernatremia. What are normal insensible losses? How does temperature affect insensible losses?**

Insensible loss averages 500 ml/day. For each 1F increase in body temperature above 100F 1000 ml of additional electrolyte free fluid is lost as sweat.

○ **T/F: Renal dose dopamine improves outcome in patients with oliguria.**

False. Renal dose dopamine increases urine output but does not improve renal function.

○ **What is normal plasma osmolality?**

Normal plasma osmolality is 285 to 295 mOsm/kg.

○   **What are some causes of hypernatremia?**

1. Diabetes insipidus (central, nephrogenic)
2. Insensible losses (burns, sweating)
3. Osmotic diuresis (mannitol, hyperglycemia)
4. Hypertonic fluid administration

○   **What are the muscular manifestations of hyperkalemia?**

Hyperkalemia partially depolarizes the cell membrane. Patients may present with neuromuscular weakness that may progress to flaccid paralysis and hypoventilation.

○   **How does acute metabolic alkalosis affect serum potassium?**

Plasma potassium falls by 0.3 mEq/L for every 0.1 unit rise in pH.

○   **How do respiratory acid-base disorders affect plasma potassium?**

Respiratory acid-base imbalances are usually not associated with significant changes in plasma potassium.

○   **What therapy is available for severe hyperkalemia?**

Calcium - protects against depolarizing effects of hyperkalemia (avoid in simultaneous digitalis toxicity)
Sodium bicarbonate - results in cellular potassium uptake
Beta-adrenergic agonists - promotes cellular uptake
Cation exchange resin - binds potassium in bowel
Loop diuretics - enhance potassium secretion in nephrons
Insulin/glucose - promotes cellular uptake
Dialysis – removes potassium from blood directly

○   **How does magnesium depletion affect potassium?**

Magnesium depletion is associated with renal potassium wasting, hypocalcemia and hypokalemia.

○   **What is the cause of hyperkalemia in diabetics?**

Cellular uptake of potassium is decreased because of hypoinsulinism. These patients often have hyporeninemic hypoaldosteronism (type IV renal tubular acidosis).

○   **What mechanism causes hypokalemia to induce a metabolic alkalosis?**

The kidney to will attempt to absorb additional potassium in exchange for hydrogen (lost from blood) in response to hypokalemia.

○   **What is the most common underlying disorder in respiratory acidosis?**

Alveolar hypoventilation.

○   **What is the daily fluid requirement for a 70 kg man?**

2500 ml/d.

❍ **At what serum sodium level would one expect to see clinical signs and symptoms of acute hyponatremia?**

Approximately 125 mEq/L.

❍ **At what sodium level would one expect signs and symptoms of hypernatremia?**

Approximately 160 mEq/L.

❍ **What are the signs and symptoms of hypernatremia?**

Restlessness, irritability, ataxia, fever, spasms and seizure.

❍ **What are the possible reasons for the development of post-operative hypokalemia?**

Intracellular shift secondary to high insulin or (-agonist levels, hypothermia, hemodilution, hyperventilation, alkalosis, on-going diuresis and nasogastric suctioning

❍ **What signs are associated with hypocalcemia?**

Decreased contractility, hypotension, ventricular arrhythmias, muscle spasms, laryngospasm, paresthesias and tetany.

❍ **What are the most common causes of hypernatremia?**

Diabetes insipidus, insensible losses, osmotic diuresis and hypertonic fluid administration.

❍ **What are the most common causes of SIADH?**

Malignancies, pulmonary disease, CNS disorders and drugs.

❍ **How fast should hyponatremia be corrected?**

No faster than 0.5 to 1.0 mEq/l/hour.

❍ **Patients with asymptomatic hyponatremia are best treated in what manner?**

Free water restriction.

❍ **Compensation for persistent hypoventilation occurs by what mechanism?**

Resorption of sodium bicarbonate by the kidney.

❍ **What is the major cause of extrarenal potassium depletion?**

Diarrhea.

❍ **What are the clinical manifestations of hypokalemia?**

Arrhythmias, muscle weakness, mental status changes, impaired intestinal peristalsis and predisposition to digitalis toxicity.

○   **T/F: Beta-blockers raise the serum potassium concentration.**

True. They inhibit uptake of potassium by skeletal muscle.

○   **What is the main determinant of the osmolarity of the extracellular fluid space?**

Serum sodium concentration.

○   **What are the most common causes of hypotonic fluid loss leading to hypernatremia?**

Diarrhea, vomiting, hyperpyrexia and excessive sweating.

○   **What are the ECG findings of a patient with hypokalemia?**

Flattened T waves, depressed ST segments, prominent U waves, arrhythmias and prolonged QT intervals.

○   **What is the quickest way to treat hyperkalemia?**

Calcium gluconate (10%) IV.

○   **What are the causes of hyperkalemia?**

Acidosis, tissue necrosis, hemolysis, blood transfusions, GI bleed, renal failure, Addison's disease, primary hypoaldosteronism, excess oral K^+ intake, RTA Type IV and medications as succinylcholine, beta-blockers, captopril, spironolactone, triamterene, amiloride and high dose penicillin.

○   **What are the causes of hypocalcemia?**

Shock, sepsis, multiple blood transfusions, hypoparathyroidism, vitamin D deficiency, pancreatitis, hypomagnesemia, alkalosis, fat embolism syndrome, phosphate overload, chronic renal failure, loop diuretics, hypoalbuminemia, tumor lysis syndrome and medications as calcitonin and mithramycin.

○   **What is the most common cause of hyperkalemia?**

Hemolysis (of lab error variety). Chronic renal failure is the most common cause of "true" hyperkalemia.

○   **In order of prevalence, what are the three most common causes of hypercalcemia?**

Malignancy, primary hyperparathyroidism and thiazide diuretics.

○   **What are the signs and symptoms of hypercalcemia?**

The most common gastrointestinal symptoms are anorexia and constipation. Remember:
Stones: Renal calculi
Bones: Osteolysis
Abdominal groans: Peptic ulcer disease and pancreatitis
Psychic overtones: Psychiatric disorders

○   **A patient with a history of alcohol abuse presents after a recent tonic-clonic seizure. What particular electrolyte abnormality should be considered and treated during evaluation?**

Hypomagnesemia.

O   **What is the most common cause of hyperphosphatemia?**

Acute and chronic renal failure.

O   **As PCO_2 increases, pH will decrease. Acutely, how much is the pH expected to decrease for every 10 mmHg increase in PCO_2?**

PH decreases by 0.08 units for each 10 mmHg increase in PCO_2.

O   **What is a better index of tissue CO_2, arterial or venous CO_2?**

Venous CO_2.

O   **Is it possible to have the identical PCO_2 in arterial and mixed venous blood?**

During respiratory arrest, pulmonary arterial blood and systemic arterial blood have the same PCO_2. However, at the tissue level, the arteriolar PCO_2 is less than that of the tissue venous PCO_2.

O   **What are treatments for respiratory acidosis?**

Intubation
Increase minute ventilation
Decrease dead space ventilation
Correct auto-PEEP (air-trapping), e.g., bronchospasm, endotracheal tube obstruction.
Treat (prevent) pulmonary embolism
Reverse muscle weakness
Reverse sedatives and narcotics
Decrease CO_2 production (shivering, hyperthermia and excess glucose load due to hyperalimentation)
Nasal CPAP or BiPAP

O   **What are the causes of high anion gap metabolic acidosis?**

The addition of strong acids to the ECF, with the exception of HCl, increases the number of unmeasured anions. Frequent causes can be remembered by the mnemonic:
M: methanol, congenital errors of metabolism
U: uremic acidosis
D: diabetic ketoacidosis
P: paraldehyde, phenformin
I: iron, isoniazid
L: lactic acidosis, D-lactic acidosis
E: ethanol, ethylene glycol
S: salicylate poisoning, solvents

O   **What are the causes of normal anion gap metabolic acidosis?**

A normal anion gap acidosis is associated with a relatively high chloride, i.e. hyperchloremic metabolic acidosis.

Gastrointestinal
Diarrhea
Following bowel preparation
High output ileal fistula or external pancreatic fistula
Ingestion of substances that bind $NaHCO_3$: e.g., cholestyramine

Renal
Proximal (Type II) renal tubular acidosis: bicarbonate wasting due to impaired HCO_3^- reabsorption; distal acidification is intact; associated with hypokalemia
Distal (Type I) renal tubular acidosis: failure of distal nephron urinary acidification; associated with hypokalemia
Distal (Type IV) renal tubular acidosis: major problem is hyperkalemia

Other
Mineralocorticoid deficiency: i.e., hypoaldosteronism
Addition of HCl acid or one of its precursors: e.g., NH_4Cl
Post-hyperventilation metabolic acidosis
Dilutional acidosis: volume infusion with high chloride containing fluids (normal saline)

O   **What is the treatment of alcoholic ketoacidosis?**

Saline infusion, glucose and thiamine.

O   **What are the causes of respiratory alkalosis (hyperventilation)?**

Hypoxemia or tissue hypoxia
Pulmonary edema
Pulmonary embolism (air, fat, thromboembolism, amniotic fluid, etc).
Shock
Cyanide toxicity
Carboxyhemoglobin
Methemoglobin
Any pulmonary parenchymal disease
Any obstructive pulmonary process

Central
Agitation, anxiety, pain
CNS infection
Central hyperventilation associated with injury to midbrain and upper pons

Metabolic acidosis
DKA
Lactic acidosis
Ingestion of acids: aspirin and alcohol

Other
Sepsis
Pregnancy
Hepatic failure
Respiratory stimulants: progesterone

O   **How should acute adrenal insufficiency be treated?**

Administration of hydrocortisone IV and crystalloid fluids containing dextrose.

O   **What are the main causes of death during an adrenal crisis?**

Circulatory collapse and hyperkalemia induced arrhythmias.

○ **What is thyrotoxicosis? What causes it?**

A hypermetabolic state occurring secondary to excess circulating thyroid hormone. Thyrotoxicosis is caused by thyroid hormone overdose, thyroid hyperfunction or thyroid inflammation.

○ **What are the hallmark clinical features of myxedema coma?**

Hypothermia and coma.

○ **What is the most important initial step in treating DKA?**

Volume replacement.

○ **What are the neurologic signs and symptoms associated with hypoglycemia?**

Hypoglycemia may produce behaviorial and neurologic dysfunction. Neurologic manifestations include paresthesias, cranial nerve palsies, transient hemiplegia, diplopia, decerebrate posturing and clonus.

○ **What laboratory finding occur in diabetic ketoacidosis?**

Elevated beta-hydroxybutyrate, acetoacetate, acetone and glucose. Ketonuria and glucosuria are present. Serum bicarbonate levels, PCO_2 and pH are decreased. Potassium levels may be elevated but will fall when the acidosis is corrected.

○ **What is the basic treatment for DKA?**

Administer fluids. Start with normal saline, switch to 0.5 normal saline, include potassium (after the patient begins to urinate and if not hyperkalemic). Give insulin, 0.1 units/kg bolus followed by 5 to 10 units/hour. Add glucose to the IV fluid when the glucose level falls below 250 mg/dl and give the patient a phosphate supplement when the level drops below 1.0 mg/dl. Religiously monitor glucose, electrolytes (including anion gap), ketones, volume status and the patient's symptoms.

○ **What are the key features of non-ketotic hyperosmolar coma?**

Hyperosmolality, hyperglycemia and dehydration. Blood sugar levels are > 800 mg/dl, serum osmolality is > 350 mOsm/kg and serum ketones are negative.

○ **What is the treatment for non-ketotic hyperosmolar coma?**

This is treated much like DKA with the caveat that the patient requires less insulin. It is important to initiate IV normal saline before giving insulin. Some suggest that an IV insulin bolus is not necessary in this condition.

○ **What is the most common precipitant of thyroid storm?**

Infection.

○ **What signs and symptoms are helpful for diagnosing thyroid storm?**

Eye signs of Graves' disease, a history of hyperthyroidism, widened pulse pressure, hypertension, a palpable goiter, tachycardia, fever, diaphoresis, increased CNS activity, emotional lability, heart failure and coma.

○   **What are some diagnostic findings of thyroid storm?**

Tachycardia, CNS dysfunction, cardiovascular dysfunction, GI system dysfunction and a temperature > 37.8° C (100° F).

○   **What is the most common cause of hypothyroidism?**

Primary thyroid failure (as opposed to secondary or pituitary etiology). The primary etiology of hypothyroidism in adults is the use of radioactive iodine or subtotal thyroidectomy in the treatment for Graves' disease. The second most common cause is autoimmune thyroid disorder.

○   **What is the most common cause of secondary adrenal insufficiency and adrenal crisis?**

Iatrogenic adrenal suppression from prolonged steroid use. Rapid withdrawal of steroids may lead to collapse and death.

○   **What pH decrease is expected with an increase of PCO_2 of 10 mmHg?**

0.08.

○   **What are the two primary causes of metabolic alkalosis?**

Loss of hydrogen and chloride from the stomach and overzealous diuresis with loss of hydrogen, potassium and chloride.

○   **What are the key therapies used to treat nonketotic hyperosmolar coma?**

Intravenous fluids and insulin.

○   **What precipitants are likely to lead to DKA in an otherwise controlled diabetic?**

Infection, cardiac ischemia, medications, lack of compliance with insulin and diet..

○   **What are usual glucose levels seen in patients with non-ketogenic coma?**

Often between 800 to 1000 mg/dl.

○   **What dangerous abdominal infections occur in diabetic patients?**

Emphysematous cholecystitis, ischemic bowel, diverticular abscess, emphysematous pyelonephritis or pyonephrosis.

○   **Diffuse abdominal pain with bloody stools and a high serum lactate in a diabetic might suggest what gastrointestinal disease?**

Ischemic or necrotic bowel.

○   **What are the signs/symptoms of hypothyroidism?**

Decreased mental acuity, hoarseness, somnolence, cold intolerance, dry skin, brittle hair and weight gain. Physical exam reveals hypothermia, generalized edema, hypoventilation, sinus bradycardia and possibly hypertension.

○ **T/F: Cardiac output (CO) is decreased in hypothyroidism.**

True.

○ **What are the causes of alveolar hypoventilation in myxedematous hypothyroid patients?**

Respiratory center depression with decreased CO_2 sensitivity, defective respiratory muscle strength and airway obstruction due to tongue enlargement.

○ **What associated laboratory abnormalities are expected in hypothyroidism?**

Hyponatremia, hypoglycemia, hypercholesterolemia and anemia

○ **What are the hemodynamic changes seen with thyroid storm?**

Tachycardia, increased cardiac output and decreased systemic vascular resistance (SVR).

○ **What are the ophthalmologic signs in hyperthyroidism?**

Exophthalmos, lid lag, lid retraction and periorbital swelling.

○ **What are the associated laboratory findings in hyperthyroidism?**

Hypercalcemia, hypokalemia, hyperglycemia, anemia, leukocytosis with a left shift, hyperbilirubinemia and increased alkaline phosphatase.

○ **What is the initial treatment of thyroid storm?**

Intravenous fluids, acetaminophen, propranolol, propylthiouracil (PTU) and iodine.

○ **What are the CNS manifestations of myxedema?**

Depression, memory loss, ataxia, frank psychosis and coma.

○ **What is the most common cause of chronic primary adrenal insufficiency (Addison's Disease)?**

Autoimmune disease.

○ **What are the most specific signs of primary adrenal insufficiency?**

Hyperpigmentation of the skin and mucosal membranes.

○ **What is the emergent steroid replacement in adrenal insufficiency?**

Hydrocortisone 100 mg intravenously every 8 hours.

○ **What patients should receive fluorocortisone?**

Those with primary adrenal insufficiency.

○ **What is the characteristic hemodynamic pattern of adrenal insufficiency?**

Decreased systemic vascular resistance and to a lessor degree, decreased cardiac contractility.

O   **A 45 year old male develops hypotension, lethargy, a hemoglobin of 12 gm/dl and a blood glucose of 34 mg/dl 24 hours after colectomy. His history is significant for a renal transplant 3 years ago. What is the most likely diagnosis?**

Addisonian crisis.

O   **What is the etiology of Cushing's disease?**

Hypersecretion of ACTH by the pituitary.

O   **What is the most common cause of acute adrenocortical insufficiency?**

Withdrawal of chronic steroid therapy.

O   **What is the possible adverse effect seen during very rapid correction of severe hyperglycemia?**

Cerebral edema.

O   **What clinical manifestations are common to all patients with Cushing's syndrome?**

Moon faces, buffalo hump, obesity, hypertrichosis, hypertension, growth retardation, easy bruising, purple striae on the hips and abdomen and amenorrhea in girls.

O   **Differentiate between non-ketotic hyperosmolar coma and DKA.**

In non-ketotic hyperosmolar coma, glucose is very high, often > 800. The serum osmolality is also very high, with average about 380. Nitroprusside test is negative.
In DKA, glucose is more often in the range of 600. The serum osmolality is approximately 350. Nitroprusside test is positive.

O   **What focal signs may be present in a patient with non-ketotic hyperosmolar coma?**

These patients may have hemisensory deficits or hemiparesis. 10 to 15% of these patients have a seizure.

O   **Which common electrolyte disturbances occur in patients who have acute pancreatitis?**

Hypocalcemia and hypomagnesemia.

O   **What are the most common causes of the hypotonic fluid loss which leads to hypernatremia?**

Diarrhea, vomiting, hyperpyrexia, and excessive sweating.

O   **What are the signs and symptoms of hypernatremia?**

Confusion, muscle irritability, seizures, respiratory paralysis, and coma.

O   **What are the ECG findings on a patient with hypokalemia?**

Flattened T-waves, depressed ST segments, prominent P-waves, prominent U-waves, and prolonged QT and PR intervals.

○ **What are the ECG findings on a patient with hyperkalemia?**

Peaked T-waves, prolonged QT and PR intervals, diminished P-waves, depressed T-waves, QRS widening, levels exceeding 10 mEq/L, and a classic sine wave.

○ **What is the first ECG finding for a patient with hyperkalemia?**

The development of tall-peaked T-waves at levels of 5.6–6.0 mEq/L, which are best seen in the precordial leads.

○ **What are the causes of hyperkalemia?**

Acidosis, tissue necrosis, hemolysis, blood transfusions, GI bleed, renal failure, Addison's disease, primary hypoaldosteronism, excess po K+ intake, RTA IV, and medications such as succinylcholine, β-blockers, captopril (Capoten), spironolactone, triamterene, amiloride, and high dose penicillin.

○ **What are the causes of hypocalcemia?**

Shock, sepsis, multiple blood transfusions, hypoparathyroidism, vitamin D deficiency, pancreatitis, hypomagnesemia, alkalosis, fat embolism syndrome, phosphate overload, chronic renal failure, loop diuretics, hypoalbuminemia, tumor lysis syndrome, and medication, such as Dilantin, phenobarbital, heparin, theophylline, cimetidine, and gentamicin.

○ **What are the most common causes of hypercalcemia?**

In descending order: malignancy, primary hyperparathyroidism, and thiazide diuretics.

○ **What are the signs and symptoms of hypercalcemia?**

The most common gastrointestinal symptoms are anorexia and constipation. A classic mnemonic can be used to remember them:

Stones: renal calculi.
Bones: osteolysis.
Abdominal groans: peptic ulcer disease and pancreatitis.
Psychic overtones: psychiatric disorders.

○ **What is the most common cause of hyperphosphatemia?**

Acute and chronic renal failure.

○ **What causes acute adrenal crisis?**

It occurs secondary to a major stress, such as surgery, severe injury, myocardial infarction, or any other illness in a patient with primary or secondary adrenal insufficiency.

○ **What is thyrotoxicosis, and what are its causes?**

A hypermetabolic state that occurs secondary to excess circulating thyroid hormone caused by thyroid hormone overdose, thyroid hyperfunction, or thyroid inflammation.

○ **What are the neurologic signs and symptoms of hypoglycemia?**

Paresthesias, cranial nerve palsies, transient hemiplegia, diplopia, decerebrate posturing, and clonus.

O   **What are the signs and symptoms of thyroid storm?**

Tachycardia, fever, diaphoresis, increased CNS activity, heart failure, coma, and death.

O   **What is another name for life-threatening hypothyroidism?**

Myxedema coma. This condition occurs in elderly women during the winter months and is stimulated by infection and stress.

O   **What are the signs and symptoms of Addison's disease?**

Hyperpigmentation, hyperkalemia, alopecia, and ascending paralysis secondary to hyperkalemia. Lab findings in Addison's disease indicate hypoglycemia, hyponatremia, hyperkalemia, and azotemia.

O   **What are the principal signs and symptoms in adrenal crisis?**

Abdominal pain, hypotension, and shock. The common cause of adrenal crisis is withdrawal of steroids. Treatment of adrenal crisis is the administration of hydrocortisone (Solu-Cortef), 100 mg IV bolus and 100 mg added to the first liter of D5 0.9 NS.

O   **What electrolyte disorder is associated with hypercalcemia?**

Hypokalemia.

O   **What changes in urine output would you expect after administering vasopressin?**

Decrease in urine output for up to 24-96 hours.

O   **Following a thyroidectomy, what nerve are you testing if you ask the patient to speak?**

The laryngeal nerve. Damage to this nerve is a potential complication following thyroid surgery.

O   **Following a subtotal thyroidectomy, you periodically slip a gloved hand behind the patient's neck. What is the rationale for this action?**

Assessment of post operative bleeding.

O   **What is the best indication that a patient with Addison's disease is receiving the correct amount of glucocorticoids?**

Daily weights as a means of detecting fluid imbalance. Rapid weight gain could indicate fluid retention and hormone replacement therapy would need to be adjusted.

O   **A physician orders sodium polystyrene sulfonate (Kayexalate). What would be the most likely reason for administering this drug?**

Elevated serum potassium level.

TOXICOLOGY PEARLS

O   **For what substances is activated charcoal is not effective?**

Alcohols, ions and acids and bases.

O   **What is the appropriate treatment for QRS widening in tricyclic antidepressant (TCA) poisoning?**

$NaHCO_3$ is administered intravenously for patients with a QRS > 100 ms $NaHCO_3$ is bolused IV and repeated until the blood pH is between 7.50 and 7.55. An infusion of $NaHCO_3$ is then continued. Potassium levels must be closely monitored.

O   **What is the appropriate treatment for TCA induced seizures?**

Benzodiazepines and barbiturates are the agents of choice. Phenytoin is not generally effective.

O   **What signs and symptoms are typical of the serotonin syndrome?**

Agitation, anxiety, sinus tachycardia, hyperthermia, shivering, tremor, hyperreflexia, myoclonus, muscular rigidity and diarrhea.

O   **What clinical findings occur with the neuroleptic malignant syndrome?**

Altered mental status, muscular rigidity, autonomic instability, hyperthermia and rhabdomyolysis.

O   **What are the signs and symptoms of lithium toxicity?**

Neurological signs and symptoms include tremor, hyperreflexia, clonus, fasciculations, seizures and coma. GI signs and symptoms consist of nausea, vomiting and diarrhea. Cardiovascular findings include ST-T wave changes, bradycardia, conduction defects and arrhythmias.

O   **What is the treatment for lithium toxicity?**

Supportive care, normal saline diuresis, hemodialysis for patients with clinical signs of severe poisoning, renal failure or decreasing urine output.

O   **What is the pharmacological treatment for alcohol withdrawal?**

Benzodiazepines.

O   **What acid-base disturbance is typical for salicylate poisoning?**

Mixed respiratory alkalosis and metabolic acidosis.

O   **What are the 4 stages of acetaminophen (APAP) poisoning?**

Stage I: 30 minutes to 24 hours, nausea and vomiting

Stage II: 24 to 48 hours, abdominal pain and elevated LFTs
Stage III: 72 to 96 hours, LFTs peak, nausea and vomiting
Stage IV: 4 days to 2 weeks, resolution or fulminant hepatic failure

○   **How is the nomogram utilized in a patient who ingests an extended relief formulation of APAP?**

4 hour and 8 hour levels are obtained (at least).

○   **What is the appropriate initial treatment of theophylline induced seizures?**

Benzodiazepines and barbiturates initially. Theophylline induced seizures warrant hemodialysis or hemoperfusion.

○   **Why is multidose activated charcoal administration advocated for theophylline poisoning?**

Theophylline undergoes enterohepatic circulation.

○   **What is the antidote for beta-blocker poisoning?**

Glucagon.

○   **What is the treatment for calcium channel blocker poisoning?**

IV calcium, isoproterenol, glucagon, transvenous pacer, atropine and vasopressors, such as norepinephrine, epinephrine or dopamine.

○   **What are the four stages of iron poisoning?**

Stage I: Initial hour: gastrointestinal symptomatology, including abdominal pain, vomiting and diarrhea
Stage II: 6 to 24 hours: quiescent period during which time iron is absorbed
Stage III: > 12 hours: shock, metabolic acidosis, hepatic dysfunction, heart failure, cerebral dysfunction and renal failure
Stage IV: 1 day to 1 week: gastric outlet or small bowel obstruction secondary to scarring

○   **What is the antidote to iron poisoning?**

Deferoxamine.

○   **What antihypertensive agent may induce cyanide poisoning?**

Nitroprusside.

○   **Under what circumstance is the use of Done's nomogram appropriate?**

Only when the patient has an acute single ingestion of a non-enteric coated ASA without recent prior use.

○   **How does N-acetylcysteine (NAC, Mucomyst) work?**

NAC enters cells and is metabolized to cysteine, which serves as a glutathione precursor. Glutathione is a free radical scavenger.

○   **What are the indications for emergent hyperbaric oxygen therapy?**

1) Loss of consciousness
2) Focal neurologic findings
3) Carboxyhemoglobin level greater that 25%
4) Myocardial ischemia
5) Pregnancy

O   **What symptoms are typical of mild to moderate carbon monoxide (CO) poisoning?**

Headache, nausea, dizziness, weakness and difficulty concentrating.

O   **How does carbon monoxide cause toxicity?**

Carbon monoxide has an affinity for hemoglobin 200 to 250 times greater than oxygen and displaces oxygen from its binding sites. It also causes a leftward shift of the oxyhemoglobin dissociation curve. These effects decrease oxygen delivery to the tissues.

O   **Delirium tremens occurs how long after the cessation of alcohol consumption?**

On average 3 to 5 days.

O   **What class of drugs is best to treat delirium tremens?**

Benzodiazepines.

O   **What is the classic triad of Wernicke's encephalopathy?**

Global confusion, oculomotor disturbances and ataxia.

O   **What is the accepted antidote for methanol poisoning?**

Ethanol administration. Patients with high serum levels or who are very ill may also require hemodialysis.

O   **What constitutes definitive therapy for moderate to severe lithium toxicity?**

Hemodialysis.

O   **What are the indications for hemodialysis in lithium toxicity?**

Serum lithium level above 4.0 mEq/l, renal failure and severe clinical symptoms.

NUTRITION MANAGEMENT PEARLS

○ **What are the goals of nutritional therapy?**

Maintain lean body mass, minimize catabolism, preserve organ function and promote immune function.

○ **When should enteral nutrition be started?**

Most proponents believe enteral nutrition should be started as soon as possible, preferably in the first 24 hours after injury or surgery (assuming no ileus).

○ **Are immunocompetence and vital organ function dependent upon nutritional support?**

Yes. Both are secondary goals of nutritional support.

○ **What is the predominant energy source used during starvation by a healthy subject?**

Lipids.

○ **What two methods are frequently used to assess nutritional status in critically ill patients?**

Indirect calorimetry and nitrogen balance.

○ **What is the goal of protein delivery?**

To achieve a positive nitrogen balance.

○ **What is the most common manifestation of excessive carbohydrate administration?**

Hyperglycemia.

○ **Can lipid emulsions be useful in patients needing volume restriction or demonstrating carbohydrate intolerance?**

Yes. Lipids are calorie dense compared to dextrose solutions.

○ **What minimum percentage of total calories should be supplied as lipid to prevent fatty acid deficiency?**

Five percent of total calories at minimum.

○ **How long does it take non-stressed patients receiving lipid-free total parenteral nutrition (TPN) to demonstrate evidence of essential fatty acid deficiency?**

Within four weeks. Hypermetabolic patients within ten days.

O   **What clinical symptoms are seen with hypophosphatemia brought on by refeeding a malnourished patient?**

Weakness and congestive heart failure.

O   **Have immunoenriched diets, containing substrates such as omega-3 fish oils, arginine and RNA nucleotides, been found to improve outcome?**

Yes, a number of recent studies suggest improvement using enteral immunoenriched formulas.

O   **What is the preferred route for the delivery of nutrition, enteral or parenteral?**

The enteral route.

O   **When should nutritional support be started?**

As soon as a hypermetabolic state (e.g., trauma or sepsis), underlying malnutrition or an expected delay in resuming an oral diet of > 5-10 days is recognized.

O   **What complications are associated with enteral nutrition?**

Complications involve routes of access to the GI tract (e.g., feeding tube displacement and obstruction), the GI tract itself (e.g., nausea, vomiting and diarrhea) or the metabolic system (e.g., hyperglycemia and hypophosphatemia).

O   **Has pre-operative nutritional support for malnourished patients been shown to be reduce post-operative morbidity?**

Yes, for those with severe malnutrition.

O   **In which patients is parenteral nutritional support indicated?**

When enteral access is unobtainable, enteral feeding contraindicated or when the level of enteral nutrition fails to meet requirements.

O   **In which patients is intravenous nutritional support unlikely to be of benefit?**

Those expected to start oral intake in 5 to 7 days or with mild injuries.

O   **Typically, what feeding route requires a greater length of time to reach full support?**

Enteral.

O   **Can lipids be given through a peripheral vein?**

Yes. They are iso-osmotic, unlike the concentrated dextrose solutions that should be infused centrally.

O   **What are the complications of parenteral nutrition?**

Those associated with catheter insertion (e.g., pneumothorax), the indwelling line (e.g., line sepsis, thrombosis), lipid emulsions (e.g., pancreatitis, reticuloendothelial dysfunction) and GI tract complications (e.g., cholestasis, acalculous cholecystitis).

O   **Can overfeeding result in difficulty weaning a patient from mechanical ventilation?**

Yes. This is related to increased energy expenditure, oxygen consumption and CO_2 production with a resultant increase in respiratory rate and minute ventilation.

O   **Can underfeeding result in difficulty weaning a patient from mechanical ventilation?**

Yes. Malnutrition can cause respiratory muscle weakness and ventilator dependence.

O   **Among protein, fat and carbohydrate, which can provide the most energy per molecule and which the least?**

Fat generates the most energy at 9 kcal/g while amino acids provide 4 kcal/g and glucose only 3.4 kcal/g.

O   **During times of glycogen depletion what source of energy is utilized by tissues that are obligate glucose users?**

Protein is the only other source of glucose. Conversion of amino acids to alpha-keto analogues allows the proteins to be used in gluconeogenesis. Lipids are highly inefficient since only the glycerol portion of the triglyceride molecule can be used for glucose synthesis.

O   **What are the major metabolic and physiologic effects of glucose, protein and fat during times of stress?**

Gluconeogenesis is increased by the liver while peripheral glucose use is reduced, resulting in hyperglycemia. Skeletal muscle undergoes increased proteolysis which can manifest as muscle wasting and increased excretion of uninary free nitrogen. Fat metabolism is also increased in an effort to decrease the amount of glucose being used.

O   **What happens to serum triglyceride, free fatty acid and glycerol levels during stress/sepsis?**

Elevated triglyceride levels and normal to elevated fatty acid and glycerol levels are seen during stress/sepsis. This is thought to be secondary to the increased lipolysis stimulated by cortisol, catecholamines and glucagon.

O   **How does worsening liver failure seen in sepsis/trauma effect the clearance of aromatic amino acids (AAAs) as opposed to branched chain amino acids (BCAAs) and what is the significance of this?**

Liver failure leads to a decreased ability to clear AAAs, a situation that does not occur with BCAAs. The excess AAAs are thought to be metabolized to false neurotransmitters which may antagonize the effects of catecholamines or cross the blood brain barrier and cause encephalopathy.

O   **What protein sparing event occurs early on in starvation?**

Early on in starvation the brain, which has the largest obligate requirements for glucose, begins to use ketones instead of glucose for energy. This reduction in the need for glucose minimizes the amount of proteolysis that is occurring.

O   **A 30 year old woman is endotracheally intubated and needs nutrition. She has a functioning gastrointestinal tract. What are the advantages of enteral nutrition when compared to parenteral nutrition?**

Enteral nutrition is more physiologic, has a trophic effect on gastrointestinal cells, avoids the need for a central venous catheter and its complications and costs less.

O   **A previously healthy 20 year old woman is injured in a motor vehicle accident. The day following admission her serum albumin is noted to be 2.8. Why is her serum albumin low?**

The decreased albumin in this patient is a marker of the injury response rather than of impaired nutrition.

O   **What happens to nitrogen reserves after trauma?**

Nitrogen reserves are mobilized due to accelerated protein catabolism.

O   **What is the maximum osmolarity of solutions that should be infused into a peripheral vein?**

Nine hundred mOsm. Parenteral nutrition solutions are commonly greater than 1500 mOsm and require central venous access for delivery.

O   **A critically ill patient's intravenous access is via a peripherally inserted central catheter (PICC). Can solutions with an osmolarity of greater than 900 mOsm be infused through a PICC?**

Yes. Although the insertion site is peripheral, the catheter tip is in a central vein and thus there is no osmolarity restriction.

O   **A 40 year old woman has had a small intestine resection. What minimum length of small bowel is required for enteral absorption of nutrients and below which parenteral nutrition must be considered?**

A minimum of 100 centimeters of small intestine is needed to sustain life.

O   **A 55 year old man is scheduled for a distal splenorenal shunt for esophageal varices. His total parenteral nutrition (TPN) solution (Hepatamine) contains less aromatic amino acids and more branched-chain amino acids than standard solutions. What is the indication for this solution?**

Hepatic encephalopathy. In hepatic failure there is an elevation of phenylalanine and methionine (aromatic amino acids) and a decrease in leucine, isoleucine and valine (branched-chain amino acids). This formula is used in an attempt to normalize plasma amino acids, based on the theory that hepatic encephalopathy may be due to this plasma amino acid change and a resulting imbalance of neurotransmitters in the brain.

O   **When total parenteral nutrition (TPN) is orderred the concentrations of what two electrolytes must be monitored to prevent precipitation?**

Calcium and phosphate.

O   **When total parenteral nutrition (TPN) is prescribed, what anions are generally used to form sodium and potassium salts?**

Chloride and acetate.

O   **What nutritional deficiency should be considered if a patient has unexplained lactic acidosis?**

Thiamine deficiency.

O   **How is lactate cleared from the blood?**

By the liver using gluconeogenic and oxidative pathways. A normal liver can remove up to 400 grams per day of lactate.

○   **What metallic nutrient may require supplementation in patients on long term total parenteral nutrition (TPN) because it is not part of multi-trace elements (MTE)?**

Iron.

○   **A patient on total parenteral nutrition (TPN) has severe diarrhea. What trace element may need to be supplemented?**

Zinc.

○   **An order is placed for multi-trace elements as "MTE-5." What five trace elements are included?**

Zinc, copper, chromium, manganese and selenium.

○   **An order is placed for multivitamins as "MVI-12." What vitamin is excluded and must be added separately to total parenteral nutrition (TPN) solutions?**

Vitamin K.

○   **The non-essential amino acid glutamine is not contained in commercial parenteral nutrition solutions. Why not?**

Because of stability and shelf-life limitations. Although the body is capable of making large quantities of glutamine, in stress states glutamine consumption exceeds production and glutamine depletion results. It is thought of as "conditionally essential" but whether or not administering glutamine improves patient outcome remains to be determined.

○   **What is the goal for calculated nitrogen balance in a critically ill patient?**

Positive 2 to 6 grams of nitrogen per day.

○   **Protein requirements are often stated in terms of nitrogen requirement. How do you determine the content of nitrogen in dietary protein?**

Grams of dietary protein divided by 6.25 approximates grams of nitrogen.

○   **What are the three categories of complications related to total parenteral nutrition (TPN)?**

Mechanical complications related to insertion of the central venous access catheter, metabolic complications and infection.

○   **A 50 year old trauma victim is started on total parenteral nutrition (TPN) and has new onset hyperglycemia. Why?**

The "diabetes of trauma" is due to a combination of inhibition of insulin secretion, increased glucagon release and reduced peripheral use of glucose.

○   **Which factor contributes more to an increase in carbon dioxide production, a high carbohydrate to fat ratio in the feeding solution or a high caloric intake resulting in overfeeding?**

A high caloric intake resulting in overfeeding.

○   **What are the untoward effects of overfeeding in a critically ill patient?**

Increased carbon dioxide production, increased oxygen consumption, fluid overload, hepatic steatosis and hyperglycemia. An increased carbon dioxide production may impede weaning from mechanical ventilation.

○   **A 45 year old man has not had adequate nutrition due to nausea and emesis for many days before total parenteral nutrition (TPN) is started. What mineral may be severely decreased during re-feeding?**

Serum phosphate. Hypophosphatemia may be associated with severe muscle weakness and a need for mechanical ventilation.

○   **What are three options for handling total parenteral nutrition (TPN) during the intra-operative period?**

Continue the TPN as ordered, discontinue the TPN by tapering over several hours during the pre-operative period or replace TPN with ten percent dextrose during surgery.

○   **During prolonged surgery, what laboratory tests should be monitored because a patient is receiving total parenteral nutrition (TPN)?**

Plasma glucose and potassium.

IMMUNOLOGY AND TRANSPLANTATION PEARLS

○ **What is an orthotopic graft?**

A graft placed in the anatomic position normally occupied by such tissue.

○ **What triggers the rejection reaction after transplantation?**

The immune response to the HLA antigens on the cells of the transplanted organ/tissue.

○ **What is the role of methotrexate in chronic immunosuppression?**

It is used clinically only for bone marrow transplantation as graft-versus-host (GVH) prophylaxis.

○ **What are the clinical uses of cyclophosphamide?**

It is used in renal transplant patients when liver toxicity prohibits the use of azathioprine and for bone marrow recipients.

○ **What side effects are specific to cyclophosphamide?**

Prompt fluid retention, severe hemorrhagic cystitis and cardiac toxicity.

○ **What are the adverse effects of cyclosporine?**

Hirsutism, neurotoxicity, hyperkalemia, nephrotoxicity, hypertension and tremors.

○ **What is the most common cause of death in transplant recipients?**

Infection.

○ **Which drugs are used most often to prevent lung rejection?**

Cyclosporine, azathioprine and corticosteroids.

○ **What are the clinical findings in acute lung rejection?**

Dyspnea, fever, hypoxemia and infiltrates on CXR.

○ **What is the typical manifestation of chronic lung rejection?**

Progressive dyspnea with decline in FEV1 (at least 20% from baseline), usually after three months.

○ **What is the most common cause of infectious complications associated with lung transplantation?**

Bacterial, which often occur early after the transplantation. Gram negative organisms are the most common.

○ **What is the most common viral infection associated with lung transplantation?**

CMV, which occurs 1 to 3 months post-transplantation.

○ **What other viral infections occur after lung transplantation?**

RSV and herpes simplex. The latter has been less common since the use of prophylactic regimens containing acyclovir or ganciclovir.

○ **Which fungal infections are the most common in lung transplant patients?**

Candida and aspergillus.

○ **When is Pneumocystis carinii pneumonia most likely to be seen in a transplant patient?**

2 to 6 months post transplantation.

○ **Fever, sternal tenderness, erythema and purulent drainage suggest what diagnosis 48 hours post-operative heart transplantation?**

Mediastinitis caused by *S. aureus*, *S. epidermidis* or gram negative bacilli.

○ **What is the most common site of bacterial infection in all types of transplant patients?**

Lung (35%).

○ **What is graft versus host disease (GVHD)?**

Engraftment of immunocompetent donor cells into an immunocompromised host, resulting in cell-mediated cytotoxic destruction of host cells if an immunologic incompatibility exists.

○ **When does acute GVHD present and what are the typical manifestations?**

Acute GVHD typically occurs around day 19 (median), just as the patient begins to engraft and is characterized by erythroderma, cholestatic hepatitis and enteritis.

○ **What is the clinical definition of chronic GVHD (cGVHD)?**

As early as 60 to 70 days status-post engraftment, the patient exhibits signs of a systemic autoimmune process, manifesting as Sjogren's syndrome, systemic lupus erythematosus, scleroderma, primary biliary cirrhosis and commonly experiences recurrent infection with encapsulated bacteria, fungi or viruses.

○ **What are significant toxic side effects of cyclosporine therapy?**

Neurotoxic: tremors, paraesthesia, headache, confusion, somnolence, seizures and coma.
Hepatotoxic: cholestasis, cholelithiasis and hemorrhagic necrosis.
Endocrine: ketosis, hyperprolactinemia, hypertestosteronemia, gynecomastia and impaired spermatogenesis.
Metabolic: hypomagnesemia, hyperuricemia, hyperglycemia, hyperkalemia and hypocholesterolemia.
Vascular: hypertension, vasculitic hemolytic-uremic syndrome and atherogenesis.

Nephrotoxic: oliguria, acute tubular damage, fluid retention, interstitial fibrosis and tubular atrophy.

○ **What conditions predispose liver transplant patients to renal failure?**

1) Hypovolemia.
2) Ascites formation.
3) Hepatorenal syndrome.

○ **On induction for lung transplantation, patients with severe chronic obstructive pulmonary disease (COPD) are often hemodynamically unstable. Why?**

COPD patients are frequently very volume depleted. On induction and commencement of positive pressure ventilation, they have a tendency to auto-peep secondary to air trapping and "breath stacking," severely reducing venous return and cardiac output. These patients should be preloaded with crystalloid and ventilated with shallow tidal volumes and a long expiratory time.

○ **In a patient needing renal transplantation list some common pre-operative problems that are often encountered?**

These problems include inadequate or excessive intravascular volume, electrolyte abnormalities, hypertension, anemia, concurrent drug therapy or complications associated with DM (cardiac and vascular).

○ **In a patient needing renal transplantation why is the hemoglobin level low?**

Chronic anemia with hemoglobin levels of 5 to 7 results from decreased production of erythropoietin and diminished red cell survival time. Iron absorption from the gastrointestinal tract may also be decreased in patients with ESRD leading to iron deficiency.

○ **In a patient who has undergone renal transplantation what are some of the early post-operative complications?**

Renal artery occlusion, hyperacute rejection, acute renal failure, graft rupture, wound infection and urinary fistula.

○ **In a patient who has undergone renal transplantation what are the signs of rejection?**

Decreased urine output, fever and increased serum creatinine. The kidney is often enlarged and tender to palpation. A renal biopsy is necessary to verify the diagnosis.

○ **What are the most common liver diseases for which liver transplantation is required?**

Chronic active hepatitis, cholestatic liver disease, biliary atresia and alcoholic cirrhosis.

○ **What are the most common causes of encephalopathy following liver transplantation?**

Gastrointestinal bleeding or other protein loads and hepatic coma secondary to cerebral edema and increased intracranial pressure.

○ **Why is adequate venous access so critical in patients undergoing liver transplantation?**

Because liver transplantation is associated with major volume losses secondary to coagulopathies.

O   **A 50 year old male, status-post liver transplant, has rapidly rising serum bilirubin and transaminases as well as hyperkalemia, hypoglycemia and coagulopathy. What is the most likely diagnosis?**

Thrombotic occlusion of the hepatic artery or portal vein.

O   **What is the appropriate treatment for the above patient?**

Retransplantation.

O   **What is the most common regimen of immunosuppression following cardiac transplantation?**

Triple therapy with oral cyclosporine, azathioprine and prednisone.

O   **What signs and symptoms are associated with cardiac rejection?**

Malaise, fatigue, dyspnea/orthopnea, tachycardia, a ventricular gallop, rales and edema.

O   **What are the indications for double-lung transplantation?**

Cystic fibrosis, bronchiectasis, pulmonary hypertension, correctable congenital defects and emphysema.

O   **What is the standard immunosuppressive management following renal transplantation?**

Cyclosporine, azathioprine and prednisone.

O   **What is the differential diagnosis for early anuria following renal transplantation?**

Hypovolemia, thrombosis of the renal artery or vein, hyperacute rejection, compression of the kidney or obstruction to urine flow.

O   **What is the treatment of choice for a patient in anaphylactic shock?**

Epinephrine intravenously.

O   **What cardiac complication commonly occurs with SLE, juvenile rheumatoid arthritis and rheumatoid arthritis?**

Pericarditis.

O   **What causes fatality in hereditary angioedema?**

Edema of the larynx.

ETHICS AND PAIN MANAGEMENT PEARLS

○ **What is a health care proxy?**

This is an individual who acts as a surrogate in making decisions regarding another individual's health care should the person become unable to do so. This is usually the spouse of the patient.

○ **What is power of attorney?**

This document declares an individual who has the legal right to make decisions regarding the health care of an individual who is unable to do so.

○ **What is a living will?**

A living will specifies that certain medical procedures (CPR, etc) not be performed in the event that the patient lacks the capacity to decline the procedures.

○ **What is an advance directive?**

This document is a living will or a durable power of attorney for health care.

○ **T/F: A patient who is fully coherent and is a Jehovah's Witness is having a massive lower GI hemorrhage. The patient is an adult and refuses blood products. The physician is legally bound to coerce the patient to receive blood because withholding it may result in the patient's death.**

False. The principle of autonomy dictates that this patient may refuse blood products even if it results in his/her death.

○ **What must be present to decide that a patient has the capacity to make health care decisions?**

The patient must have knowledge of the options and their consequences and an understanding of the costs and benefits of the options relative to a set of stable values.

○ **T/F: A patient who refuses a recommendation by their physician is incapacitated to make health care decisions.**

False.

○ **T/F: A patient with stage I bronchogenic carcinoma has pulmonary edema requiring mechanical ventilation. You explain this to the patient and he agrees with proceeding with intubation and mechanical ventilation. His wife refuses. The physician should not intubate the patient.**

False. The principle of autonomy declares that each individual is the ultimate arbiter of his or her own health care.

❍   **May a physician be found liable for a child's reaction to a vaccine she/he administers?**

Only if a typical reasonable competent physician would not have acted as the physician did.

❍   **Is there an ethical difference between withholding and withdrawing life-support measures in patients with acute respiratory failure?**

Ethical principles underlying the decision to withhold intubation and mechanical ventilation apply equally when patients or proxies request discontinuance of care for patients who have no hope for an acceptable and meaningful recovery.

❍   **How do opioids affect the respiratory pattern?**

Decrease in rate, tidal volume and minute ventilation. The pattern may also be irregular.

❍   **Which anesthetics when combined with opioids can lead to cardiovascular depression?**

Nitrous oxide, volatile anesthetics, propofol and barbiturates.

❍   **What are some of the common side effects of opiates and their treatments?**

Side effect	Treatment
Nausea	Phenothiazines, metoclopramide
Sedation	Naloxone
Constipation	Laxatives, stool softeners
Urinary retention	Reduction of dosage, catheterization
Pruritis	Diphenhydramine, naloxone
Respiratory depression	Naloxone

❍   **Why are IM injections of opioids a poor choice for post-operative analgesia?**

Variable blood levels, unpredictable absorption, delayed onset, lag to peak analgesic effect and pain. PCA administration eliminates these problems.

❍   **What are the major advantages of epidural opioid administration?**

Improved pain relief, steady pain relief, decreased post-operative morbidity, improved pulmonary function and shortened hospital stays.

❍   **What are the signs of impending epidural opioid toxicity?**

Altered mental status, decreased level of consciousness, oxygen desaturation, decreased respiratory rate, miosis, increased CO_2 levels.

❍   **What are the major contraindications to the use of NSAIDs in the post-operative period?**

Recent history of GI bleed and ulcers, severe insensitivity to the NSAIDs, impaired renal function and any significant hematologic abnormality that might predispose to bleeding.

❍   **What are the effects of NSAIDs and aspirin on platelet function?**

All NSAIDs produce reversible inhibition of platelets. Aspirin produces irreversible platelet function. The effects of the NSAIDs persist until the drug is mostly eliminated. Those with longer half-lives have an increased incidence of complications as well.

○ **When might it be advantageous to use epidural over IV PCA medication in the post-operative period?**

Upper abdominal, vascular and thoracic surgeries benefit from epidural analgesics.

○ **What are the disadvantages of using opioid agonist/antagonists or partial agonists in post-operative pain?**

These agents have a ceiling effect on analgesia above which there is no benefit to analgesia with increased dose. Above this ceiling effect these agents have adverse psychomimetic effects and other adverse effects. These agents are not as potent analgesics as conventional opioid agonists.

○ **With what procedures has epidural analgesia been shown to be particularly beneficial?**

Procedure	Benefit
Thoracotomy	Pulmonary function
Joint replacement	Decreased DVT, earlier ambulation
Vascular procedures	Improved blood flow, patency
Pediatric cardiac	Decreased ventilator time and hospital stay
Abdominal surgery	Earlier return of bowel recovery

○ **What is the best way to manage post-operative pain in the patient with a current problem of illegal opioid abuse and addiction?**

"PRN" injections are to be avoided. After a thorough and frank discussion about the pain and expectations about pain relief the patient should receive adequate doses of either scheduled oral or IV opioids or preferably, IV PCA with a background infusion. Consideration must be made for the patient's tolerance to "usual" doses of opioids. Larger bolus doses should be anticipated. Adjunct analgesics such as NSAIDs may be appropriate.

○ **What are commonly encountered side effects of epidurally administered local anesthetic infusions?**

In large quantities a partial sympathetic block may precipitate hypotension, particularly orthostatic hypotension. With more dilute concentrations this is avoided. Mild motor or sensory loss may occur. Urinary retention, particularly in the very young or the elderly male patient, may occur.

○ **What are the major physiologic adverse effects of uncontrolled post-operative pain?**

System	Adverse Effect
Gastrointestinal	Ileus
Cardiovascular	Increased sympathetic effect (BP, Pulse) and angina
Pulmonary	Atelectasis, hypoxia, shunting and CO_2 retention
CNS	Altered mental status and stress
Immunologic	Impaired wound healing

BIBLIOGRAPHY

BOOKS/ARTICLES

Plantz, SH. *Emergency Medicine Pearls of Wisdom,* 6th ed., McGraw-Hill; 2005.

Advanced Trauma Life Support Student Manual, 7th ed., Chicago: American College of Surgeons; 2002.

Albert, DM. *Clinical Practice Principles and Practice of Ophthalmology,* Vol. 2. Philadelphia: W.B. Saunders Co.; 1994.

American College of Surgeon's Committee on Trauma. *Advanced Trauma Life Support Manual,* 7th ed., Chicago: American College of Surgeons, 2002.

Arieff, A. & Defronzo, R. *Fluid, Electrolyte and Acid Base Disorders,* 2nd ed. New York: Churchill Livingstone; 1995.

Auerbach, PS. *Management of Wilderness and Environmental Emergencies,* 4th ed. St. Louis: CV Mosby Company; 2001.

Baer, C. Clinical Pharmacology and Nursing, 3rd ed. Springhouse PA: Springhouse Corp., 1996.

Bakerman, S. *ABCs of Interpretive Laboratory Data,* 4th ed. Greenville: Interpretive Laboratory Data, Inc; 2002.

Barash PG, Cullen BF, Stoelting RK (eds): *Clinical Anesthesia,* 4th ed. Philadelphia: Lippincott-Raven; 2000.

Barkin, RM. *Emergency Pediatrics,* 6th ed. St. Louis: CV Mosby Company; 2003.

Barie PS, Shires GT (eds): *Surgical Intensive Care.* Boston: Little, Brown and Co.; 1993.

Bayley, E. A Comprehensive Curriculum for Trauma Nursing. Boston: Jones & Bartlett Pubs, Inc., 1992,

Berhman, RE & Vaughn, VC. *Nelson Textbook of Pediatrics,* 17th ed. WB Saunders Company; 2004.

Berkow, R. *The Merck Manual,* 17th ed. Rahway: John Wiley & Sons; 2004.

Bradley, WG. *Neurology in Clinical Practice.* 4th ed., Newtown: Butterworth-Heineman; 2003.

Catalano, J.T. Critical Care Nursing Certification, 1st ed. Pennsylvania: Springhouse Publishers; 1995.

Civetta JM, Taylor RW, Kirby RR. *Critical Care,* 3rd ed. New York: Lippincott-Raven Publishers; 1997.

Clochesy, J.M. Critical Care Nursing, 2nd ed. Philadelphia: W.B. Saunders Co., 1996.

Cullom, RD Jr. *The Wills Eye Manual: Office and Emergency Room Diagnosis and Treatment of Eye Disease,* 4th ed. Philadelphia: JB Lippencott Co.; 2004.

Ellenhorn, MJ. *Ellenhorn's Medical Toxicology: Diagnosis and Treatment of Human Poisoning,* 2nd ed. Baltimore: Williams & Wilkins; 1997.

Feliciano DV, Moore EE, Mattox KL (eds): *Trauma,* 3rd ed. Stamford: Appleton & Lange; 1996.

Fishman, AP. *Fishman's Pulmonary Diseases and Disorders,* 3rd ed. New York: McGraw-Hill; 2002.

Fitzpatrick, TB. *Color Atlas and Synopsis of Clinical Dermatology.* 4th ed., New York: McGraw-Hill Publishing Company; 2000.

Flomenbaum, N. *Emergency Diagnostic Testing,* 2nd ed. St. Louis: Mosby-Year Book, Inc.; 1995.

Fontaine, K.L., Essentials of Mental Health Nursing, 3rd ed. Redwood City, California: Addison-Wesley, 1995.

Fuhrman, BP & Zimmerman, JJ. *Pediatric Critical Care.* 2nd ed., Mosby-Year Book, Inc.; 1997.

Goldfrank, LR, et al: *Goldfrank's Toxicologic Emergencies,* 7th ed. Stamford: Appleton & Lange; 2002.

Hall JB, Schmidt GA, Wood LDH. *Principles of Critical Care,* 3rd ed. New York: McGraw Hill, 2005.

Harris, JH. *The Radiology of Emergency Medicine,* 4th ed. Baltimore: Williams and Wilkins; 1999.

Harrison, TR. *Principles of Internal Medicine,* 16th ed. New York: McGraw-Hill Book Company; 2004.

Harwood-Nuss, A. *The Clinical Practice of Emergency Medicine,* 3rd ed. Philadelphia: JB Lippincott Company; 2001.

Hickey, J. The Clinical Practice of Neurological and Neurosurgical Nursing. 5th ed. Philadelphia: J.B. Lippincott Co., 2002.

Holland, JF. *Cancer Medicine,* 4th ed. Baltimore: Williams & Wilkins; 1997.

Kaplan, HI. *Comprehensive Textbook of Psychiatry,* 8th ed., 2004

Kelley, WN. *Textbook of Internal Medicine,* 3rd ed. Lippincott-Raven; 1997.

Koenig, K. *Clinical Emergency Medicine.* New York: McGraw-Hill; 1996.

Lenhardt, R. *Pulmonary Pearls of Wisdom.* Watertown: Mt. Auburn Press; 1998.

Levin, DL & Morris, FC. *Essentials of Pediatric Intensive Care.* 2nd ed., Matthew Medical Books, Inc.; 1997.

Mandell, D & B. *Principles and Practice of Infectious Diseases,* 5th ed., Churchill Livingstone, 2000.

Marino, P. *The ICU Book,* 2nd ed. Baltimore: Williams and Wilkins; 1998.

Miller, RD (ed): *Anesthesia,* 5th ed. New York: Churchill Livingstone; 2000.

Murray, JF and Nadel, JA (ed): *Textbook of Respiratory Medicine,* 3rd ed., Philadelphia: WB Saunders; 2000.

Nelson, W.E. *Textbook of Pediatrics.* 17th ed., Philadelphia: W.B. Saunders Company; 2004.

Peitzman AB, Rhodes M, Schwab CW, Yealy DM (eds): *The Trauma Manual.* Philadelphia: Lippincott-Raven; 1998.

Physicians' Desk Reference, 59th ed. Oradell: Medical Economics Company Inc; 2005.

Plantz, SH. *Emergency Medicine PreTest, Self-Assessment and Review.* McGraw-Hill; 1990.

Plantz, SH. *Emergency Medicine.* Baltimore: Williams & Wilkins; 1998.

Reese, RE & Betts, RF (eds): *A Practical Approach to Infectious Diseases*, 4th ed. Boston: Little, Brown and Company. 1988.

Roland, L. *Merritt's Textbook of Neurology.* 10th ed., Williams & Wilkins; 2000.

Rosen, P. *Emergency Medicine Concepts and Clinical Practice,* 4th ed. St. Louis: Mosby Year Book; 1998.

Rowe, RC. *The Harriet Lane Handbook,* 16th ed. Chicago: Year Book Medical Publishers, Inc; 2002.

Schrier, RW & Gottschalk, CW. *Diseases of the Kidney*, 7th ed. Boston: Little, Brown and Company; 2001.

Shapiro BA, Kacmarek RM, Cane RD, et al: *Clinical Application of Respiratory Care,* 4th.ed. St. Louis: Mosby-Year Book, Inc.; 1991.

Shapiro BA, Peruzzi WT, Templin R. *Clinical Application of Blood Gases*, 5th ed. St. Louis: Mosby-Year Book, Inc.; 1994.

Simon, RR. *Emergency Orthopedics: The Extremities,* 2nd ed. Norwalk: Appleton & Lange; 1987.

Simon, RR. *Emergency Procedures and Techniques,* 4th ed. Baltimore: Williams and Wilkins; 2001.

Squire, LF. *Fundamentals of Radiology,* 6th ed. Cambridge: Harvard University Press; 2004.

Stedman, TL. *Illustrated Stedman's Medical Dictionary,* 27th ed. Baltimore: Williams & Wilkins; 2000.

Stewart, CE. *Environmental Emergencies.* Baltimore: Williams and Wilkins; 1990.

Textbook of Neonatal Resuscitation. American Heart Association; 2002.

Textbook of Pediatric Advanced Life Support. Dallas: American Heart Association; 2003.

Textbook of Pediatric Advanced Life Support. American Heart Association; 2003.

Tietjen PA, Kaner, RJ and Quinn CE: Aspiration Emergencies. *Clinics in Chest Medicine* 1994;15:117-135.

Tintinalli, JE. *Emergency Medicine A Comprehensive Study Guide,* 6th ed. New York: McGraw-Hill, Inc; 2003.

Thelan, L.A. Critical Care Nursing: Diagnosis and Management, 4th ed., St Louis: Mosby Year Book; 2001.

Townsend, CM. *SabistonTextbook of Surgery: The Biological Basis of Modern Surgical Practice.* 17th ed., Philadelphia: W.B. Saunders Company; 2004.

Urban, N. Guidelines for Critical Care Nursing. St Louis: Mosby Year Book, Inc. 1995.

Wagner, GS & Marriott, HJL. *Practical Electrocardiography,* 10th ed. Baltimore: Williams and Wilkins; 2001.

Weigelt, JA & Lewis, FR (eds): *Surgical Critical Care.* Philadelphia: WB Saunders Co.; 1996.

Weiner, HL. *Neurology for the House Officer,* 4th ed. Baltimore: Williams & Wilkins; 1989.

Werber, SS & Ober, KP. Acute adrenal insufficiency. *Endocrinol Metab Clin North Am.* 1993; 22:303-28.

West, JB. *Respiratory Physiology: The Essentials*, 6th ed. Baltimore: Williams & Wilkins; 2000.

Wilson, JD & Foster, DW. *Williams Textbook of Endocrinology*, 10th ed. Philadelphia: W.B. Saunders; 2002.

Wilson, R & Walt, A. *Management of Trauma: Pitfalls and Practice*, 2nd ed. Philadelphia: Williams & Wilkins; 1996.

Winn, RH. *Youmans Neurological Surgery.* 5th ed., Philadelphia: W.B. Saunders; 2003.

Zevitz, M. *Cardiology Pearls of Wisdom*. Watertown: Mt. Auburn Press; 1999.

Zevitz, M. *Internal Medicine Pearls of Wisdom*. Watertown: Mt. Auburn Press; 1998.